THE MUSCULOSKELETAL SYSTEM

Differential Diagnosis from Symptoms and Physical Signs

John McM. Mennell, MD
Clinical Professor
Department of Physical Medicine and Rehabilitation
College of Osteopathic Medicine
Michigan State University
East Lansing, Michigan

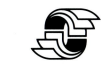

AN ASPEN PUBLICATION®
Aspen Publishers, Inc.
Gaithersburg, Maryland
1992

Library of Congress Cataloging-in-Publication Data

Mennell, John McM. (John McMillan), 1916 —
The musculoskeletal system : differential diagnosis from symptoms and
physical signs / John Mennell.
p.   cm.
Includes bibliographical references and index.
ISBN: 0-8342-0255-7
1. Musculoskeletal system—Diseases—Diagnosis.
2. Musculoskeletal system—Examination.
3. Diagnosis, Differential. I. Title.
[DNLM: 1. Bone Diseases—diagnosis. 2. Diagnosis, Differential.
3. Joint Diseases—diagnosis. 4. Muscular Diseases—diagnosis.
5. Musculoskeletal System—physiopathology. WE 141 M547m]
RC925.7.M36   1991
616.7'075—dc20
DNLM/DLC
for Library of Congress
91-4866
CIP

The authors have made every effort to ensure the accuracy of the information herein.
However, appropriate information sources should be consulted, especially for new or
unfamiliar procedures. It is the responsibility of every practitioner to evaluate the
appropriateness of a particular opinion in the context of actual clinical situations and
with due consideration to new developments. Authors, editors, and the publisher
cannot be held responsible for any typographical or other errors found in this book.

Editorial Services: Barbara Marsh

Library of Congress Catalog Card Number: 91-4866
ISBN: 0-8342-0255-7

Printed in the United States of America

2 3 4 5

Table .of Contents

Foreword

I met John Mennell in 1966 when I spent an academic year at the University of Pennsylvania Graduate School of Medicine and he was Chief of Physical Medicine and Rehabilitation (PM&R) at Philadelphia General Hospital. William Erdman, M.D., Professor and Chief of PM&R at the University of Pennsylvania, introduced him to our class of eager and "oh so smart" senior orthopaedic residents saying, "I am not sure what this man does, but he is the best darned diagnostician of musculoskeletal disease I know." An actor in his youth in England, John Mennell made theatrical presentations that enthralled his listeners. However, we were captured by what he said, not how he said it. He introduced us to the concept of the mechanical body as a system, with the whole being qualitatively different from that of the sum of its individual parts. His alarmingly simple concepts are self-evident and indisputable: that all joints in the body are mechanically similar, just local adaptations of a grand design, and that widely accepted simple mechanical principles can be applied to mechanical structures.

Simple mechanical malfunction, loss of "play" movement ("play" being present in every mechanical thing that moves) was theorized as the source of "mechanical" rather than "pathologic" impairment of the joint. Why not? Are there not "functional" impairments of the gastrointestinal system, genitourinary system, cardiac and respiratory systems, in which there is no demonstrable pathology? In modern parlance,[1] "dynamical diseases" (disease of the dynamics of the system) belong to the new science of "Chaos,"[2] the science of complex dynamical systems such as the weather, ecology, and living matter. Chaos deals in non-linear mathematical events that are extremely sensitive to initial conditions. Local hot spots, such as the eruption of Mt. St. Helen's, may have global consequences in the weather; a minor local event, such as the introduction of Dutch elm disease to North America, ends up wiping out the entire elm tree population; and a small variation of a gene can create a major somatic change. Along those lines, minimum loss of joint play can affect the gross movement of the joint, and in turn, total body movement.

I followed Doctor Mennell through the rest of the year and learned more about seeing, touching, and understanding body mechanics in a few short months than I had in my previous eight years of training. Over the years, as I have taught with him and read and re-read his writings and listened to his lectures, I have continued to gain new insights with each encounter. Over and over again, I have tested his theory of joint play and have found no exception to the rule.

In this book, Doctor Mennell organizes his years of work in a single work. His work is as up to date as the 90s and at the same time, it is delightfully old-fashioned. The information and concepts are updated and are as new and as fresh and important today as when they were first presented. The theme is old fashioned in that it celebrates the skills of a physician in physical diagnosis, listening to the patient, touching and understanding the body systems, and relegating new state-of-the-art technologies to an adjunct position. After all, experience tells us that what is state of the art

technology today will be superseded by newer and better machines that prove present day technology inadequate. The mind and the hand are unlikely to be replaced in the foreseeable future.

This book will be read and enjoyed but not then put aside. It will become a reference work to be read and re-read over and over again.

Stephen M. Levin, MD, FACS

REFERENCES

1. Glass L, MacKay MC. Pathological conditions resulting from instabilities in physiological control systems. *Annals of the New York Academy of Sciences.* 1979; 316:214.

2. Gleick J. *Chaos: making a new science.* New York, NY: Viking Penguin Inc.; 1967.

Preface

After 38 years of experience specializing in the field of musculoskeletal medicine, I was asked by Aspen Publishers, Inc. to pull together all that I have written into the system in which it belongs. This should have been done years ago. Had that been the case, the tail would not be wagging the dog.

I have acknowledged everything I quote of others' work and writing where appropriate. Otherwise the work and writing are mine. For the most part it has been published here and there in English; some of it has been published in Japanese and Spanish. Please refer to the bibliography at the end of this book.

The format of this product is designed to be "why and when" to do a procedure, rather than "how" to do a procedure. Therefore, all the topographical areas of the musculoskeletal system are not represented. Chapter 5 uses the foot, the low back, and the wrist and hand as examples of clinical examination.

In the past two or three years innumerable books on the subject of back pain have been published. They all address pain in the musculoskeletal system; none of them address the differential diagnosis of any one structure in the musculoskeletal system which, because of a pathological change, is giving rise to the symptoms. In medical school too little stress is laid on the fact that there is no function of the body that can take place without some part of the musculoskeletal system being used. Death denotes cessation of function of the musculoskeletal system. We cannot eat or excrete without using some part of the system; we cannot communicate without using some part of the system. Muscles guard against pain arising from any structure in the system, including the muscles themselves. The confusing point, however, is that they react the same way regardless of the structures from which the pain originates.

This book concerns problems of the neglected musculoskeletal system. The main difficulty with this is that it is not possible to study this system with the usual research tools available to allopathic medicine. Everything in this system is concerned with living and ceases in death. Investigators are not equipped to study living structures in either health or mechanical dysfunction. Note the inclusion of the word *mechanical*. Mechanical pathology is a new concept to most practitioners of the healing arts. So far as we know, there are no changes at the cellular level in mechanics, and it seems unlikely that there are because relief of symptoms on restoration of normal mechanics is immediate. There may be biochemical changes and neurovascular changes associated with mechanical dysfunction; these could be immediately reversible.

Second, all impairments in the musculoskeletal system are associated with symptoms of pain and loss of movement to some degree or another. With mechanical impairment on clinical examination, there are tissue texture changes, asymmetry of anatomic posture, changes in architecture, and movement to be found; and loss of movement to be appreciated. We have not yet adequately settled the question as to whether we treat pain or loss of movement by our mechanical treatment, which we call manipulation.

Third, it must still be recognized that, on clinical examination, while looking for mechanical or disease signs, there are two barriers from normalcy to alert the examiner to a musculoskeletal problem. First, there is a barrier of pain that precludes full movement; and second, there is a barrier of loss of movement that may or may not be associated with pain. Usually, when pain is a predominant feature of disability, its relief is associated with restoration of movement. Alteration of joint movement can be assessed by palpation or feeling, in which skills most lack training. It can also be assessed by performing passive manipulative examining movements, which require just as much skill but in which most are untutored. A simple clinical fact is that the lighter your touch the more you feel.

Fourth, it is necessary to recognize that there is mechanical play between moving parts of any moving structure built into the joint to ensure its efficient functioning. Freedom of all joint play movements, which almost invariably are all less than ⅛ inch in range *within* the joint, is a prerequisite to normal functional movement. If play is impaired or lost, function is impaired and cannot be restored until play is first restored. As play movements in the body are not under the control of muscles and cannot be produced by specific muscle action or by exercise play can only be restored by passive movement induced by a mechanic—the therapist. Joints will only move in the way they wish in planes that are predetermined by their anatomy. To try to force any movement in any other manner or plane is simply creating damage. The

normal range of play movements at every synovial joint has to be learned. One must also learn that the mechanic attends to each synovial joint in any topographic area and never attacks the area itself. Thus any reference to any topographic area in therapy is absolutely contraindicated. Spinal manipulative therapy is meaningless. One never therapeutically manipulates a wrist, a foot, a knee, an ankle, a shoulder, an elbow, a hand, a hip, or the spine; one manipulates a joint or each joint in any given topographic area after detecting loss of joint play in it by using manipulative examining techniques designed to demonstrate normal play.

Fifth, we have to learn to recognize that a normally functioning musculoskeletal system is essential and prerequisite to health in all the other body systems. If pain from loss of joint play, which we call joint dysfunction, is unrelieved, it soon becomes somatic dysfunction by somatovisceral reflex mechanisms. To this must be added the effect of psychologic trauma from unrelieved pain from any source, be it somatic, visceral, or stress and tension.

The acquiring of information is the beginning of learning; knowledge develops once information is acquired. With this work we have to try to develop the wisdom needed for the successful use of this knowledge. Once it is obtained, wisdom is universal; it belongs to all. So please let us avoid putting names of people to techniques, and please let us avoid getting sidetracked into any prejudiced or biased discussions. It must be obvious that every skilled therapist in the area of manual medicine and manual therapy must, in the long run, be doing the same thing to the same thing to achieve the same results. To discuss schisms is to backtrack to the discussion of information. We are here to go forward and, it is hoped, to acquire wisdom.

Editor's Note: Should you be interested in purchasing video tapes illustrating the Diagnosis and Treatment Using Manipulative Techniques for: **The Upper Extremities** (25 minutes), **The Lower Extremities** (20 minutes), **The Low Back** (32 minutes), **The Cervical and Thoracic Spine** (32 minutes), **Spray and Stretch for Pain and Muscle Spasm** (33 minutes); please contact the Physical Medicine Research Foundation, 207 West Hastings St., Suite 510, Vancouver, BC, V6B 1H7, Canada. FAX (604) 684-6247.

Acknowledgments

The passage of time is inescapable. Often it is somewhat unkind. After 50 years of writing, suddenly it dawned on me that my holographic skills have greatly deteriorated—a most unhappy state of affairs. But the fickle hand of fortune brought Mary Phelan and later David Priddy into my orbit. Their incredible interest in my work, which developed almost against their will, initiated the process that has brought this manuscript to see the light as a published product, as it should be and is.

The people to whom I am indebted for the production of this book are many indeed. Each knows his or her contribution and will, I trust, accept my thanks anonymously and my apology if I fail to name every individual who deserves credit.

Although neither has disclosed the details to me, I believe that I was approached by Aspen Publishers at the urging of Dana Lawrence, editor of the *Journal of Manipulation and Physiological Treatment*, who prompted Martha Sasser, an Acquisitions Editor with Aspen, to offer me a contract without any foreknowledge of my work. I wish to thank both of them for their trust.

Once signed, Loretta Stock took over the process. She suffered through seemingly endless delays as deadline after deadline passed. I wish to thank her for her unusual patience.

Dr. Janet G. Travell, who has been my longtime devoted friend, has given me permission to use any of the artwork she produced over the years. Only pictures prepared by her can adequately depict her work. I owe a very special debt to my friend Thomas Shaw, who very kindly consented to put together the clinical observations which form the basis of the "Forward Head Syndrome" section in Chapter 6. In my experience, never has anyone expressed him- or herself better on this subject. Tom has done a wonderful job in clarifying such a complicated subject, and for that I thank him.

Because I live in a rural community, I ran across an unexpected problem in producing a publishable text—finding part-time help to assist me. I had six secretaries, none of whom had medical experience, but all of whom were more than willing to dive into this work. Especially, my thanks are due to Martha Linker, who rapidly became a friend of the family. My very special step-granddaughter, Dorée, was my pinch hitter, pulling me out of my more desperate moments. Tammie Huff came to the rescue as my final helper when the page proofs arrived. Thank you, Tammie.

Shawn Angell is a medical illustrator who has given up the profession but came back to it to provide new illustrations for this book. My model, Tim Page, is a very quiet person, one of the greatest assets that a model can have. Thank you, Tim. Jason Cane, who is at the beginning of his career, produced the new line drawings, which skillfully highlight the important aspects of what he illustrates.

As patient as everyone has been with me, no one was taxed more than my devoted wife. She had no idea when this project began what it would mean to be married to an author. Thank you, Betty.

Had there not been incredible motivation and love shown by everyone who pitched in to help, the book would not have been produced. They all knew and appreciated the undeniable fact that they were contributing to a work which many might consider to be on the fringes of orthodoxy. My readers will soon realize that this is not the case. They will learn that I am just trying to fill an educational gap which has been overlooked for too long. My hope is that this book will be able to serve a need that plagues our patients, and as such will be a service to our profession.

J. McM. M.
Advance, North Carolina

chapter 1

Introduction

This work addresses the problem of differential diagnosis of the causes of symptoms arising in and from the Cinderella of the body systems that bring patients into the offices of physicians in ever increasing numbers as they seek relief.

The following quotation is taken from a contribution to the *London Times* by Mr Pearce Wright, its Science Editor, and highlights the need:

> "Britain is becoming a Nation of Pain in the Necks," according to studies prepared for the Arthritis Rheumatism Research Council. At any given time, more than 10% of adults are experiencing some discomfort in the neck, with or without associated arm pain. Shoulder complaints rank fifth among rheumatic conditions as the cause of incapacity and visits to the doctor. Doctors report an increasing number of people coming to see them with pain in the neck and shoulders but there is no obvious explanation for the increase. Sufferers are right to seek help because more aid now can be given with the recent advances in diagnosis and treatment. We are generally better at diagnosis so we can decide whether the pain is temporary and will go away with a little [care] or whether there is an underlying cause like arthritis which needs more serious attention. The good news for most people is if they have a painful shoulder it is not arthritis of the joint but inflammation around it.

The treatment of pain is not the practice of medicine; were that the case, then all that potential patients need to do is sit in front of their television sets and watch the pharmaceutical commercials. Nor is the practice of medicine an exercise in high-tech knowledge and skill. We should remember that a person must program a computer before it can become a useful tool in everyday living.

The successful practice of medicine is still based on arriving at the correct diagnosis of the cause of each patient's symptoms; this is still dependent on listening, observing, feeling, and thinking. The result of thinking is enhanced by experience: No computer is able to touch. The lighter you touch, the more you feel. Observation is the function of many human capabilities that a computer cannot possess; parenthetically, not everyone can be trained or train himself or herself to be as good an observer as everyone else. Listening is also an art that requires training, patience, experience, and, above all, wisdom. No computer has any of these advantages, nor does the filling out of a form in any way substitute for keen analytic listening.

The musculoskeletal system, which is by far the largest system in the body, has never yet been properly defined. Consequently, its ills have not been completely studied. Perhaps because it is so commonplace for it to be involved in activities of all phases of normal life, and because nature provides adequate natural healing processes, those who practice the healing arts are taught only to pay scant attention to those who complain of pain that seemingly arises from within the system. Patients who do not get well either are called noncompliant or are said to have a psychologic overlay.

Pain is just a symptom of some attack on the integrity of some structure of the system. The complicated thing about the musculoskeletal system is that pain may arise from any one of its structures and also that disease in any structure in any other of the body systems may have its symptoms and signs referred to an area of the musculoskeletal system. In such cases our brains are unable to unscramble the signals, and the musculoskeletal system reacts as though the pain in fact were arising in it.

There can be few physicians who are unaware that the symptoms of coronary occlusion may include left shoulder pain, left arm pain, and left jaw pain. Any of these pains may be severe enough to mask the less obvious symptoms that could and should draw a physician's attention to the cardiovascular system in looking for their source. If that were all, the practice of medicine might not be too difficult. Nevertheless, besides the musculoskeletal system's manifestations of cardiovascular system disease, abdominal pain may be its presenting feature. Many cardiac patients have initially been treated as though the cause of their pain were arising from a source of illness in the gastrointestinal system.

Before getting involved in any one system of the body, students of medicine should examine what a system is, and they should have more than a passing acquaintance with all the body systems.

The system is a complete entity; it is made up of its own structures, whose functions are interrelated and interdependent. At no time should it be fragmented for study; when its construction or one of its functions is interfered with, then something else in the system is stressed. If this is neglected, then chronic changes occur. From this there may be a spill-over, directly or indirectly, into any other system.

No one structure of a system can have its own identity. If only one member of a system is identified, its symptoms usually cannot be relieved until attention is paid to the whole system. Further, there can be no exception to a whole system: It is hierarchic. If an exception is found, there is no longer a system. It is, therefore, a truism that the study of a system cannot be attended by the study of fragmented areas of it. Yet fragmentation of the musculoskeletal system is an everyday occurrence when physicians look at patients whose chief complaints seemingly arise from it.

Concurrently, it is widely accepted that the weight-bearing joints of the lower extremities are in some way different from the functional joints of the upper extremities. It is only in recent years that the facet joints of the spine have been afforded any recognition at all. Ever since this recognition has been accepted, it has just as clearly been determined that these joints in the lumbar spine are somehow different from those in the cervical spine, and scant attention, if any, is paid to these joints in the thoracic spine, let alone the costovertebral joints. Such an approach vitiates the system and simply adds to the current consternation and confusion that perpetuate ignorance.

It is a time-honored dogma to those who specialize in the other body systems that pain should not be treated until its cause has been identified. The word *identified* is chosen in preference to *diagnosed* because it includes the need to determine which structure in the system is being attacked as well as what pathologic condition is attacking it. These two things must be identified before successful therapeutic endeavors can be undertaken. Nor can pain be usefully researched. It is there to draw attention to a cause that must be unveiled before it can be researched, after which one may expect that the pain is going to be resolved in a predictable manner.

chapter 2

The Musculoskeletal System

The musculoskeletal system has two equally important functions. The first is movement, and the second is support (or containment). The most important part of its movement function is perhaps that its absence is associated with death. As movement becomes more and more impaired, the functions of the systems that the musculoskeletal system is designed to contain cannot be maintained, and these other structures themselves become dysfunctional. This in itself contributes to and may hasten the final loss of function of the contained systems.

STRUCTURES OF THE MUSCULOSKELETAL SYSTEM

There are seven structures that make up this system. These structures may be affected by five generic types of pathologic states. Every structure is not affected by them all, however. If they were, it would be common sense to believe that there are 35 possible differential causes of pain symptoms. To arrive at the proper conclusion, it is logical simply to cross-match these structures with the pathologic changes.

Of the seven structures, four are sensitive and three are insensitive. The following three are insensitive:

1. *Bone.* Bone itself is insensitive, but its periosteum and endosteum are highly sensitive. Pressure or injury from outside or within the bone may cause what apparently is bone pain.
2. *Hyaline cartilage.* Hyaline cartilage is insensitive, and radiographic changes imputed to it can have no bearing on pain from it unless it is so worn away that the endosteums of the articulating bones are rubbing on each other.
3. *Fibrocartilage.* Fibrocartilage is insensitive. Interarticular menisci occur in only five joints in the body. They cannot be primary sources of pain. Although intervertebral discs are not intraarticular in the spine, they act as menisci in that movement of the synovial joints at the level of disc injury is blocked. It should be remembered that there are no intervertebral discs on either side of the first cervical vertebra.

The remaining four structures are sensitive:

1. *The synovial capsule*. The joint capsules are highly sensitive structures, and they may be a source of pain.
2. *Muscles*. The muscles are highly sensitive structures. In the diagnostic area it should be remembered that there is the fleshy part of the muscle, the tendinous part of the muscle, and in some areas tendon sheaths. Pain may arise from changes in any of these parts.
3. *Ligaments*. Ligaments are extremely sensitive structures and may be the source of pain.
4. *Bursae*. Bursae are sensitive structures and may well be the source of pain. Anatomically there are no bursae in the back. Even so, adventitious bursae may develop between "kissing" vertebrae in the lumbar area and beneath the scapula where it rubs over the angles of ribs 4, 5, and 6.

Some may be critical that the structures of the system are limited to seven. They may ask "What about the nerves?" One must accept that question, but its answer involves a discussion about the neuromusculoskeletal system. Others may ask "What about blood vessels?" This question is acceptable also, but then the discussion involves the cardiovascular-musculoskeletal system. It should be unnecessary to add these two things because the discussion would then be unending. Surprisingly, no one ever asks about the lymphatic system because attention to this system is so vital when one comes to considering therapy in the recovery phase.

Following this line of thought, some might also have questions about the skin and the fascia. These different systems must be addressed when assessing the overall status of the patient. For example, consider the emphysematous patient. Usually the pulmonary system is considered primarily at fault, followed quickly by changes in the cardiovascular system. Few observers note the tightness of the body envelope of these patients; the skin is so tight that this alone makes breathing difficult. Few draw attention to the brittleness of these patients' bones or to the loss of movement in the facet joints or the costovertebral joints in their thoracic spines. These individually may be sufficiently pain producing to limit a patient's breathing, even if it were otherwise possible.

PATHOLOGIC CAUSES THAT MAY ATTACK THE STRUCTURES

There are five broad generic categories of pathologic changes that may affect the seven structures of the musculoskeletal system: trauma, inflammation, metabolic disease, neoplasms, and congenital anomalies.

Trauma

When dealing with the musculoskeletal system, it is useful in one's diagnostic analysis to recognize that trauma should be divided into two categories: extrinsic and intrinsic. Extrinsic trauma implies multiple injuries. There is another obvious difference between extrinsic and intrinsic trauma. Invariably extrinsic trauma is associated with bleeding. It may be severe. Intrinsic trauma to joints that results in primary joint dysfunction is usually indirect and may not be associated with bleeding or any other sign of inflammatory change. There is functional impairment without structural change. Muscles may be involved in intrinsic trauma. There may be muscle fiber tears and ruptured tendons, and these may cause minor bleeding. In the back, avulsion of a transverse process is evidence of severe muscle trauma rather than bone trauma. Patients who have an avulsion fracture do not have broken backs, and this should never be conveyed to them.

Avulsion fractures may also occur in other areas. A blow or a fall onto the tip of the shoulder may result in avulsion of the greater tuberosity of the humerus or a tear in the rotator cuff. The greater trochanter of the femur may be avulsed. Adolescents indulging in excessive muscle pull, usually in sports, may avulse the epiphysis of the iliac crest (hip pointer) or the lesser trochanter of the femur (groin pull). During bone growth, epiphyseal separation may occur after an injury. A slipped epiphysis of a femoral head is not uncommon and seems to appear insidiously.

Inflammation

It should be remembered that anything that causes an inflammatory change anywhere in the body may cause musculoskeletal manifestations. The etiologic factor in inflammation anywhere in the system may arise from bacteria or bacilli, be they Gram positive or Gram negative. Inflammation can arise from parasitic infestation, serum sickness, cardiovascular diseases, tuberculosis, and infection with amebae. It can arise from spirochetes, diseases such as gout, infections such as viruses, and infections that may occur from yeasts. It even can arise from the autoimmune system diseases and blood diseases. Infection of the system may be direct, through local portals of entrance, or indirect, from distant portals of entrance: then the infection is blood borne.

Metabolic Disease

Bone is the only structure from which pain may arise when metabolic disease is the cause of pathologic change. Aching and fatigue are commonplace, but not pain. In the most simple classification of metabolic disease of bone only three entities are considered, the commonest of which is osteoporosis senilis. This must be differentiated from the more serious ones: osteomalacia and osteitis fibrosa cystica. There are other diseases that clinically appear to be the primary cause of bone pain, such as multiple myeloma, sickle cell anemia and other causes of bone infarcts, and Paget's disease.

Neoplasms

Neoplasms in any structure of the musculoskeletal system may be primary benign or malignant or secondary and metastatic. Malignant neoplasms of bone, especially in children, are particularly lethal. If treatment is to be successful, early diagnosis is essential. Pain that awakens a patient at night and appears to be coming from the musculoskeletal system should always suggest to the diagnostician the presence of a bone tumor. If this night pain is relieved by aspirin, the presence of an osteoid sarcoma may be suspected.

Congenital Anomalies

Congenital anomalies should present little difficulty in the differential diagnosis of musculoskeletal pain. One must remember, however, that often an anomaly seen on a radiograph or image is not the source of symptoms, especially pain.

One of the commonest diagnosable sources of pain arising in the musculoskeletal system is the Travell trigger point. One of its characteristics is that the patient seldom has any idea where the source of the pain is located. For the most part, the source is a long distance away from the area of pain that the patient describes.

CROSS-MATCHING STRUCTURES AND PATHOLOGIC CONDITIONS

Having established the seven structures of the musculoskeletal system and the five pathologic conditions that may affect any one of these structures, it is sensible to cross-match the structures of the system with the pathologic conditions. From this clinical exercise, it should be possible to arrive at an elective diagnosis of the pathologic condition and its location. It behooves the clinician to undertake a treatment that predictably produces relief of the patient's symptoms in a predictable time and manner.

In previous publications I have chosen to use the shoulder and the elbow as examples of this suggested clinical exercise. Because I am stressing that we are dealing with a system rather than topographic parts of the body, here I have decided to use the foot and ankle as examples. Probably there are few adults in the shoe-wearing population of the world who do not suffer from foot discomfort. The complaints range from tired feet through aching feet to frankly painful feet. In teaching about the feet and demonstrating physical examination procedures, I always insist that students use only one foot of the person on whom they are working. One cannot help it if the examining procedures being used become manual therapy procedures that predictably relieve joint dysfunction when it is present. Everyone who wears shoes immobilizes one or another, if not all, of the joints of the feet. Joint play and its loss as a cause of pain are discussed in Chapter 3. Immobilization is one of the etiologic factors that give rise to loss of joint play.

Bone, Periosteum, and Endosteum

Trauma

Any subcutaneous bone can have its periosteum bruised by direct trauma. With healing, extravasated blood organizes and adherent scar tissue forms. This produces a painful periosteal scar, which is one of the more difficult pain conditions to treat successfully. When the endosteum is subject to pressure, this results in pain. This may occur as a heralding feature of bone neoplasms, bone infections, and bone disease.

Usually when one puts bone and trauma together, the answer comes up fracture. Many fractures are not detectable by routine X-ray examination, and the physician is faced with what we call occult fractures and stress fractures. Traumatic epiphyseal separations and greenstick fractures may be caused in children by trauma during the growing years.

The common locales of occult fractures are the surgical neck of the humerus, the neck of the femur, the head of the radius, the waist of the carpal navicula, and the waist of the talus. The common locales of stress fractures are the neck of a metatarsal bone, the calcaneus (foot pain), the lower third of the tibia, the lower third of the fibula (ankle pain), the neck of the fibula (ankle pain and sometimes knee pain), a vertebral body (back pain), a rib (chest wall pain), and the hamate (wrist pain, especially in golfers).

It is not necessary to have an X-ray examination to demonstrate a fracture, nor is it necessary to rely on expensive high-tech methods of examination. Long bone has the property of the conduction of sound. If the clinician listens for this on percussion and the sound on the injured side is less than that on the uninjured side (or even absent), it is evidence of the loss of cortical continuity of the bone from whatever cause. After the healing of a fracture, the bone conduction of sound returns.

Clinically, in detecting a small bone fracture, if aspiration of blood from a hematoma localized to the seat of injury reveals fat floating on the blood, like oil on water, this is pathognomonic of the presence of a fracture.

In the foot and around the ankle, there are many areas of subcutaneous bone where local trauma can cause painful scarring once healing has taken place. This is more likely to happen in the foot when a patient unaccustomed to going about barefooted does so. The sesamoid bones, having no periosteum, are consequently spared from this. This is true of every sesamoid bone throughout the system.

Attention has been drawn to two locales in the foot where stress fractures may occur: the neck of any metatarsal bone and the waist of the talus. Callus is a late radiographic feature of a metatarsal fracture. This differs from the clinical appreciation of stress fracture of the calcaneus. If one draws a line through the long axis of the talus and another through the calcaneus, these lines intersect at an angle of about 35° on a lateral X-ray film. In the presence of an occult fracture of the calcaneus, the angle subtended by these lines is greatly reduced; indeed, the lines may become almost parallel.

In occult fracture through the waist (neck) of the talus, exquisite pain is elicited on palpation through the sinus tarsi that is too intense to be caused by any other injury. Osteochondritis juvenilis and aseptic necrosis occur in the bones of the foot. Osteochondritis occurs in the tarsal navicula (Köhler's disease) and in the head of the second metatarsal bone (Freiberg's disease). Changes in a sesamoid bone also may produce great pain and disability. The pathologist's report in such cases may leave some doubt as to whether the pathologic condition is osteochondritis or chondromalacia. Another cause of intense pain apparently from bone is Sudeck's bone atrophy, which occurs in the bones of the feet and hands. This may follow trauma that may be quite minor. Immobilization of the foot for some other reason also may cause this.

Inflammation

Any bone of the foot may become the seat of hematogenous osteomyelitis of pyogenic or granulomatous etiology. The bones may become infected by direct means when the inflammation is associated with a compound fracture or a puncture wound.

Neoplasms

The bones of the feet may become the seat of primary malignant or benign tumors and sarcomas.

Metabolic Disease

Metabolic disease of bone is a pain-producing condition, and the bones of the feet may be affected as part of the generalized disease process. Because changes in the feet may be a part of acromegaly, pain in the feet may be the presenting symptom of this condition secondary to a pituitary tumor.

Congenital Anomalies

Congenital anomalies of the bones of the feet, especially in relation to the navicula, the talus, and the calcaneus, cause painful spastic flat feet. The congenital conditions of prehallux may be a cause of pain. Morton's atavistic foot is the basis of pain from faulty weight bearing caused by the congenital anomaly. Occasionally there is an extra ossification center at the base of the fifth metatarsal bone and behind the talus. These may avulse and be the cause of pain.

Hyaline Cartilage

Trauma

Hyaline cartilage, having no nerve supply, cannot itself be the seat of pain. If it is worn away or destroyed and bone is left rubbing on bone, however, then pain ensues because endosteum rubs on endosteum. Chondral fractures may occur in joints. The only changes one can note in radiographic studies of joints that concern hyaline cartilage draw attention to the loss of joint space, which is indicative of an injured or degenerated structure.

Those who deal in radiology tend to draw attention to the loss of joint space and hypertrophic or cystic bone changes that appear around the joint margins. In the knee joint they may draw attention to the loss of joint space in either the medial or the lateral compartments, which is said to be characteristic of a meniscal injury. In the back a loss of a normal lordosis of the vertebrae in the lumbar or cervical spine is said to be characteristic of muscle spasm. This is not true.

The word *arthritis* is so abused both by lay and professional people that it is difficult to discuss the disease in any rational way. The word *arthritis* is a convenient but meaningless way of communicating with patients and purveyors of pharmaceutical products. It may become a little more meaningful as different prefixes are added. The commonest of these is *osteo*. It surely must be apparent that a patient may have pain-free osteoarthritis today and painful osteoarthritis tomorrow. It is the hope of the therapist to produce freedom from pain for the patient. Were the joint reexamined radiographically after the pain is relieved, the changes of bone in and around the joints are exactly the same, and the size of the joint space has not altered. Even with a prefix, arthritis does not necessarily become meaningful as a cause of a patient's symptoms. The pain must be arising from some other structure that has yet to be determined.

The Synovial Capsule

The joint capsules have an outer parietal fibrous layer and an inner secretive layer, which is concerned with the presence of changes in the synovial fluid. Normal synovial fluid is a distillate of blood. Its viscosity changes in trauma and disease. Among other things, its stickiness increases as it ceases to circulate in the normal way. It is from detritus of hyaline cartilage that the viscosity of the fluid is determined because of its assistance in producing hyaluronidase.

The visceral layer of the capsule is crenated (pleated) rather than smooth. If crenations are adherent to one another, the stagnant fluid between them becomes stickier. This is one explanation for adhesive capsulitis.

There is usually a capsular excess in normal joints. This is particularly seen in the glenohumeral joint, in which the excess has special anatomic recognition; it is called the subscapular bursa. It is not a bursa, however. The misnomer leads to clinical confusion and therefore unpredictable treatment. In the knee joint there is a similar excess. It is called the suprapatellar pouch. This designation does not define a clinical entity. In the facet joints of the lumbar spine there is a relatively large amount of excess capsule, which can be demonstrated by air arthrography. This excess can interpose itself between the facets. Then it is mistakenly identified as a meniscoid. The hypothesis is that when the meniscoid is pinched back pain results.

There has been some discussion about there being a meniscoid in the radio-humeral joint (hence "tennis elbow") and the acromioclavicular joint. These speculations do not fit the system. Capsular injury (ie, structural change) is associated with pain. If there is no such structure there cannot be pain from it.

Trauma

Joint dysfunction, joint subluxation, and joint dislocation occur on an ascending scale, depending on the force that is imparted into the joint by the trauma. The severity of joint reaction is in relation to the amount of injury sustained by the capsule. Joint dysfunction has been explained as impaired function of a joint without structural change. Subluxation is, by definition, a partial dislocation. This means structural change with a relatively minor degree of synovitis developing. Dislocation means disruption of the joint with severe traumatic synovitis ensuing, often with bleeding and sometimes with rupture of the capsule.

Inflammation

Excess intracapsular synovial fluid does not cause an inflammatory reaction in the joint. Blood or pus does. Foreign bodies or intraarticular fractures also set up an inflammatory reaction within the joint.

There is an unusual condition that affects synovial capsules; it is called pigmented villonodular synovitis. It is one cause of spontaneous bleeding into a joint. It is locally invasive but not metastatic. The only other condition that produces spontaneous bleeding in the joint is hemophilia.

Other conditions such as gouty crystals or crystals of pseudogout set up capsular inflammation. Many diseases produce inflammatory changes in the capsules of joints. These include gonorrhea, syphilis, granulomatous infections, collagen vascular diseases, allergic disease, serum sickness, and parasitic infestation. Joints may be involved in conditions such as ulcerative colitis, acromegaly, and other endocrine disorders. There can scarcely be a medical disease that does not have some such musculoskeletal manifestation.

Metabolic Disease

There are no metabolic diseases that involve the capsules of joints; therefore, metabolic diseases do not have to be included in the differential diagnostic survey of causes of musculoskeletal pain.

Congenital Anomalies

There are no congenital anomalies that affect synovial joint capsules, so that they do not have to be included in the differentiation of causes of musculoskeletal pain.

Neoplasms

There are both benign and malignant neoplasms arising from the synovium. The malignant synovioma is especially lethal, and it does not have to be located within a joint. Because one can never palpate a normal synovial capsule, it should be clear that if a capsule can be palpated then there is either disease or a tumor.

Ligaments

Ligaments are a common seat of pain from joints. It must be remembered that normal ligaments are never tender on palpation unless the ligament itself is injured or unless something is wrong with the joint that the ligament supports. This is true throughout the system. In the back, one must recognize that tenderness in any of the complex of supraspinous-interspinous ligaments is indicative of something wrong at an intervertebral junction rather than in any specific joint.

Trauma

Ligaments may be stretched (strained) by trauma, ligamentous fibers may be torn, or a ligament may be ruptured.

In the foot there is one discrete ligament of the subtalar joint that is palpable at the base of the sinus tarsi. Tenderness here indicates a source of pain from the subtalar joint as opposed to the mortise joint. Each of these joints is involved in a different function. The subtalar joint hurts on walking downhill, the mortise joint hurts on walking uphill, and each joint has its own range of joint play movement.

Another ligament presents a problem on palpation because its surface anatomy is usually not presented correctly. The superficial fibers of the medial collateral ligament of the knee insert into the anteromedial aspect of the tibia four fingerbreaths below the plateau of the tibia under the pes anserinus. There are four other structures inserting into the bone at this point, all of which have to be differentiated from each other. These structures are the tendons of the sartorius, the gracilis, and the semitendinosus muscles; there is also an anserinal bursa. The point is that tenderness four inches below the tibial plateau may indicate that there is a pathologic condition within the knee joint.

Other Pathologic Causes

In considering ligaments, there is no need to consider metabolic disease, tumors, or congenital anomalies in the differentiation of sources of pain. A ruptured ligament is probably a more serious injury than a fracture. The diagnosis is advanced by demonstrating abnormal, excessive movement on physical examination, which can be proved by using stress radiographs. Figure 2-1 shows tracings from radiographs of an ankle. The establishment of the diagnosis of a ruptured ligament is so important that infiltration of the injured

ligament with local anesthetic should be done to mask the pain symptoms during the procedure. If ligament healing is delayed the joint still may not resume its function, and surgical stabilization of such a joint may be indicated.

It should always be possible to define a ligament of any joint through knowledge of surface anatomy. In the back there is a palpable ligament at every junction, from the occiput down to the sacrum, behind the sacroiliac joints, in front of the sacroiliac joints (per rectum), and at the sacrococcygeal junction.

Muscle

It should be common sense that neither chemicals nor the empirical use of physical therapy affects physical disabilities in any predictable or special ways. Unless one knows the properties of the modality used and what is expected of it, such modalities are being abused. Just as sick muscles are suffering from altered physiology that can

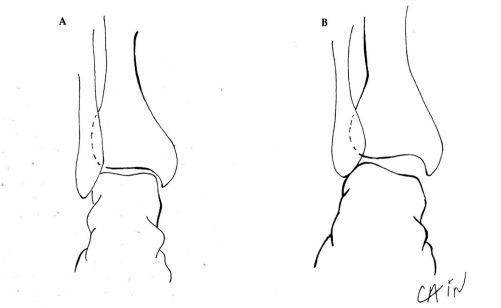

Fig. 2-1. Tracings from X-ray pictures of an ankle. (**A**) Normal, unstressed view. (**B**) Effect of stress in tilting the talus in the mortise away from the tibia. This is diagnostic of a ruptured deltoid ligament.

only be redressed by knowing their normal physiologic expectations, so a knowledge of the normal anatomy is needed to detect their sickness from the surface of the body by palpation.

Trauma

The reaction of muscle to trauma depends on whether the fleshy part of it or the tendinous part of it is involved. Contusion from extrinsic trauma is usually obvious in terms of its cause and effect. It is manifested by tenderness, swelling, and discoloration. Crushing is a special type of contusion; the wringer injury in children is a special example of this. It is becoming more rare as old-fashioned washing machines are disappearing.

Any crushing injury must be treated as a potentially lethal emergency. Neglect of such a patient in the early stages may result in Volkmann's ischemic contracture, which certainly may lead to a useless extremity and occasionally to the loss of the limb. Besides the wringer injury of the arms of children, in industrial accidents involving crushing and after stress injuries (overuse injury) the pathologic changes are commonly seen in the anterior and posterior compartments of the lower leg.

When interstitial bleeding takes place in the musculoskeletal system, its resolution results in fibrosis. This militates against successful rehabilitation because muscle layers may mat. This is frequently seen after back and knee surgery. This interferes with normal muscle action, function, and strength. Myositis ossificans is another potential and more serious complication of bleeding. Resolution of blood within joints may result in true intraarticular adhesions.

Avulsion of bone as seen in the back, the shoulder, and the foot should be looked on and reported as an injury of the muscle attached to the bone that is involved. If the separation of the avulsed fragment of the greater tuberosity of the humerus is greater than ⅛ inch, surgical reduction and fixa-

tion should be considered the desirable therapy. The greater and lesser trochanter of the femur may also be avulsed.

Inflammation

Fleshy parts of muscle may be directly involved in boils, carbuncles, pressure sores, accidental and surgical wounds, and so on. No one questions the hematogenous etiology of the spread of infection to bones, joints, muscle, and the epidural space.

Hematogenous infection brings up the question of fibrositis, which may be localized or widespread and may give rise to sudden acute pain or long-standing chronic pain. Around this diagnosis a bitter war has been waged among physicians. There has been a myriad descriptive diagnostic name changes, none of which suggests any pathologic entity that does affect muscle. There have been at least eight synonyms in diagnostic use in the past 50 years; the following come to mind: acute fibrositis, acute fibromyositis, acute myositis, fibromyalgia, polymyalgia, rheumatica, psychogenic rheumatism, and even Bornholm's disease (epidemic myalgia).

Before Travell so clearly defined the myofascial trigger point (Chapter 6), this large group of patients was included under the umbrella diagnosis of fibrositis. The differentiation is quite clear. The trigger point patient is seldom aware of the location of the trigger point causing the pain symptoms. In contrast, the fibrositis patient localizes the source well. Recognizing the pattern of referred pain from a trigger point, the clinician can predictably localize the source and draw the patient's attention to it. If the examiner then irritates the source by palpation, predictably it worsens the symptoms (or reproduces the pain pattern of which the patient is complaining). Fibrositis gives rise to no predictable patterns of pain and is found in no particular place in any muscle. Therapy that so predictably relieves patients of trigger point pain, be it acute or chronic, brings no relief to a patient with fibrositis.

One hears little these days of parasitic infestation of muscles. It must occur, but it seems to be lost in the plethora of somatic changes. There are rheumatoid nodules in collagen vascular diseases. Recently, the diagnosis eosinophilic myalgia has surfaced. One wonders whether this laboratory finding might not be overlooking the association with the blood change seen in heavy metal poisoning.

The trigger point can most easily be explained by referring to the facts that are known in the basic sciences. The structural changes giving rise to predictable symptoms most nearly coincide with medical understanding.

One of the hallmarks of life in this century, whether one is rich or poor, is that the muscles of the body are especially abused (or maybe underused), resulting in multiple microtrauma to their fibers in whatever part of the body is being misused. This results because of our frenetic way of life.

Protective guarding or muscle spasm that protects any other structure in the system adds to overuse and disuse. Both these things deprive muscle of its pumping properties. This results in a build-up of catabolites within the affected muscle(s). It also results in interference of the flushing of the system by the circulatory system. Among other things, the lymphatic system stagnates. The relaxation phase of the physiologic requirements of muscle function is lost. A vicious circle of cause and effect sets up a climate for muscle morbidity to occur. Microtrauma results in microfibrosis. The catabolite build-up itself sets up low-grade inflammatory changes in the already damaged tissue.

Let us now take an excursion into another system: the mouth. Oral hygiene is sadly deficient in the average patient. Consider an abscess at the root of the tooth or pyorrhea in the gums. It is well accepted that pressure on the jaws from biting, chewing, or even grinding of the teeth at night produces episodes of transient bacteremia. As each bacterial globus passes along its way, it is innocuous to a normal person unless it lights on some injured tissue, such as microscars from microtrauma in a muscle that is already in a morbid state. A low-grade inflammatory reaction is set up, and pain ensues. This further aggravates the already impaired muscle function, and painful areas of muscle induration become apparent to the clinician.

There may be a constant drain of infected material from a chronically infected sinus. Then there is a constant drain of infected material being swallowed with the saliva. This makes its way into the gastrointestinal system. If, as is quite common, such a patient has any degree of achlorhydria, the bacteria are not overcome and may enter the circulatory system without doing any damage until they find some less than normal tissue, frequently in the musculoskeletal system. There they set up an area of inflammation, which is the fibrositic nodule or induration that the clinician can recognize.

This is the story of autogenous intoxication. This is the common story of fibrositis secondary to some focus of infection. Commonly the sources are the teeth, tonsils, sinuses, stomach, gallbladder, appendix, and the large intestine. These days patients are not asked about these things when seeking relief of severe musculoskeletal pain that may be local or diffuse. Removal of the source is a prerequisite of successful treatment by any modality of physical therapy. Even then, one must seek for aggravating circumstances, such as sleep deprivation, lack of relaxation, poor nutrition, or any cause of fatigue that may be environmental or psychologic as well as physical. All these things, if present, should be treated, not by chemicals, but by physical and psychologic therapy.

There are two etiologic factors that produce primary fibrositis: exposure of a part of the body to cold, and any viral infection. The treatment of the first is to remove the source of the cold; the treatment of the second is to await the resolution of the viral infection. Usually there are no overt residual symptoms.

Muscle Tendons

Muscle tendons react somewhat differently from the fleshy part of muscle, and this may well be the reason for their having a different type of sensory receptor: the Golgi apparatus. The fleshy muscle has the spindle apparatus. When we come to the synovial capsule it is governed by the Ruffini apparatus.

Tendons are affected by trauma and tend to rupture instead of tearing. In the foot, the Achilles tendon and the plantaris tendon are common locations for this injury. The latter is more common from intrinsic causes than extrinsic ones.

Inflammation of tendons is moot, and clinical observation has to be the basis for the diagnosis of tendinitis. Clinically the changes of tendinitis are quite different from the inflammatory changes seen in the fleshy muscle. The changes of tendinitis occur at the musculotendinous junctions. To be able to arrive at this diagnosis, one has to be well acquainted with surface anatomy so that one can positively separate an individual musculotendinous junction as a source of pain.

The musculotendinous junction of the supraspinatus muscle is one example of this. It is situated in a hole bounded by the spine of the scapula inferiorly, the acromion process laterally, and the outer end of the clavicle anteriorly. Palpation into this hole with the tip of the index finger may produce tenderness. The patient is now asked to abduct the upper arm, which movement the examiner resists. The pain under the palpating finger gets worse. The only structural change is that tension has been exerted on the supraspinatus muscle at its musculotendinous junction, which the examiner's finger is stressing.

Another example of a musculotendinous junction as a cause of pain is the short head of the biceps. The thumb of the examiner is placed one thumbbreadth below the coracoid process of the scapula in the deltopectoral groove. If this elicits tenderness, the patient is then asked to lift the hand with the forearm supinated toward the face. This movement is resisted by the examiner. Increased pain must be coming from the musculotendinous junction of the short head of the biceps. The long head of the biceps is not usually affected by this condition, but it commonly ruptures.

Tendinitis is found at the musculotendinous junction of the biceps at the elbow. In the back this tendinitis is a common cause of pain arising from the musculotendinous junction of the sacrospinalis muscle as it joins its common tendin, which inserts into the sacrum. In the foot the musculotendinous junction of the flexor hallucis longus is particularly but not exclusively prone to tendinitis.

There is a generalized fibrositic condition found in sufferers from back pain called panniculofibrositis. Skin rolling is tight and tender all over the upper half of the back; the hyperemia generated by it is intense, and the pain is excruciating. It is most commonly found in women but is certainly not exclusive to them. The etiology of this condition is environmental as well as physical.

Pathologic Fibrosis

Just as fibrositis must be differentiated from trigger point, so it must be differentiated from pathologic fibrosis. When elastic fibers in soft tissue are lost, they do not regenerate but are replaced by fibrous tissue. This is the basis for contracture that may affect fascia, tendons, intermuscular septa, and interstitial tissue.

This also is the basis of intracapsular adhesions secondary to hemarthrosis or pyarthrosis. Painful muscle spasms must not be mistaken for painful contracture. It is virtually impossible to stretch or lengthen pathologic fibrotic tissue. Interstitial matting may occur in the abdominal wall, in the chest wall, and after surgical procedures in the back and knee.

Pathologic fibrosis is the basis for Dupuytren's contracture in the hands and feet, contracture of the plantar fascia in Perone's disease, contracture of the Achilles tendon, and tightness of the iliotibial bands.

Tendon Sheaths

In different areas of the body there are tendon sheaths around tendons, and it is important to differentiate the structure from which the pain is arising. It is important to determine whether tenosynovitis is traumatic because the condition may herald disease. There are two disease states in particular that may affect tendon sheaths: tuberculosis and collagen vascular diseases. The condition may arise from overuse of the muscle tendon, whose sheath then reacts to trauma. In such a case, the history may be masked because the patient may overlook intrinsic overuse trauma.

The differentiation can be made by palpation. When the muscle is passively moved, the palpating finger of the clinician not only elicits pain but also feels crepitus if the tendon sheath is at fault. Sometimes it is possible to do a differential nerve block because tendon sheaths usually have a different nerve supply from the tendon within.

Neoplasms

Neoplasms of muscle are not common, yet they are often malignant and may be of mixed type. Benign neoplasms of tendon sheaths such as giant cell tumor and xanthoma may be found. Tendon sheaths can be the seat of malignant neoplasms. These neoplasms are more likely to cause a functional disturbance than pain. They should not be too difficult to diagnose because most patients can recognize an unexpected lump or bump.

Metabolic Diseases

Metabolic diseases of muscle are usually benign. Frequently there is more of an aching in the muscle during exercise.

Congenital Anomalies

Muscles are sometimes absent at birth. As growth occurs, however, substitution for an absent muscle takes place, and no pain results from this. Consequently, the lack of muscle does not have to be considered in the differential assessment.

Fibrocartilage (Menisci and Discs)

There are only five joints in the body in which intraarticular menisci are found. In themselves they are probably not pain producing because they have no sensory nerve supply. Even so, when they are injured or loosened or are involved in another pathologic condition, be it inflammatory or disease, they lock up joints and produce capsular pain. The joint play of these joints is lost, and manipulative therapy may indeed be the treatment of choice to relieve the resulting disability.

The joints in which there are menisci are the following: the sternoclavicular joint, the ulnatriquetral joint, the knee joint (in which of course there are two), the temporomandibular joint, and the radiohumeral joint. Authors of anatomic textbooks are at odds as to whether there is a meniscus in the acromioclavicular joint, but it is certainly not constructed to contain one.

The intervertebral disc, although not intraarticular, acts as though it were. When injured it acts as though it were intraarticular and blocks or locks the synovial joints at the junction of the injury to the disc, usually unilaterally on the side of the radiating pain. There is no anatomic reason for anyone to suffer pain in the back just because there is a prolapsed disc in the epidural space. The back pain can only arise from loss of joint play in the facet joint at the level of injury. This is seldom attended to during treatment for the disc itself. The affected joint in the back is often relieved by restoration of its normal play.

Inflammation

Inflammatory conditions do not primarily affect menisci, but after any inflammatory process has resolved in the joint in which it is situated the meniscus may be loosened at its attachment and may become involved in pain-producing dysfunction.

Metabolic Disease

Pseudogout and ochronosis may affect menisci and cause internal derangement of the affected joint.

Neoplasms

There are no neoplasms that primarily affect menisci, so that they do not play a part in the differential diagnostic evaluation of causes of musculoskeletal pain.

Congenital Anomalies

The only congenital anomaly of a meniscus involves the lateral meniscus in the knee. This may be discoid instead of semilunar and may cause blocking of the joint, resulting in pain. Parenthetically, the lateral meniscus of the knee suffers pseudomucinous degeneration after injury, whereas a similar injury to the medial meniscus may result in a fracture of it. This is probably because the lateral meniscus is anchored in front and behind, whereas the medial meniscus has a third anchor beneath the medial collateral ligament.

Bursae

It should go without saying that a patient cannot suffer from bursitis in a place where there is no anatomic bursa. Bursitis has become a lay term for any pain that appears to be coming from the shoulder. There are no anatomic bursae in the back, but adventitious bursae may develop. They may be found under the vertebral border of the scapula, where it rubs over the angles of ribs 4, 5, and 6. Adventitious bursae can also develop between vertebral spinous processes in the lumbar spine if they should impinge on one another from backward bending.

To make a diagnosis of bursitis, the source of pain must be at a place where it is known that there is a bursa; at that location there must be a palpable swelling, which may be warm or hot to the touch. It is fluctuant, probably discolored, and tender.

Trauma

Inflamed bursae will only hurt if they are tightly distended. The olecranon bursa, when it is swollen, distends its synovium limply and just hangs like a bag from the back of the elbow. If a patient leans on the elbow, of course, it is going to hurt, but hurting is different from having a musculoskeletal pain. It is easily relieved by not leaning on it.

The coronoid bursa is small. When swollen it is visible on top of the lacertus fibrosus on full extension of the elbow. This is acutely painful. The bursa disappears when the elbow flexes. The condition is easily overlooked.

Unless it is clear that a bursa has been affected by trauma, the pain from bursitis more often heralds the onset of disease such as gout or collagen vascular disease.

Inflammation

Traumatic inflammatory bursitis of the ischial bursa and the greater trochanteric bursa at the hip is frequently diagnosed, and yet there is on examination no physical sign of an inflamed bursa. These pains more often arise from Travell's trigger points in the quadratus lumborum muscle. These establish themselves after injuries to the lower back.

Metabolic Disease

There are no metabolic diseases that affect bursae. They do not therefore enter the differentiation of the causes of musculoskeletal pain.

Neoplasms

One must assume that there may be neoplastic changes that affect bursae, but they must be rare. Bursae are lined with a synovial lining.

Congenital Anomalies

There are no congenital changes in bursae on record, so that this cause of musculoskeletal pain does not have to be included in the differential diagnostic survey.

chapter 3

After Structural Diagnosis

When the structure has been identified as the source of symptoms, there are further decisions to be made. The differential diagnosis must be pursued before elective treatment is undertaken, which should have a predictable result. There are two important words in diagnostic medicine that are used rather indiscriminately: *acute* and *chronic*. Both words may be used in relation to time or in relation to the degree of pathologic change.

The onset of a bad abdominal pain is acute both in time and in regard to the pathologic state that is causing the symptoms. The onset of pain heralding many conditions initially may be insidious and may cause a patient mild and intermittent discomfort. In describing the chief complaint, the word *chronic* (in this instance) is more apt than *acute*. A patient who has undergone surgery for an acute pain and postoperatively has the same pain is usually designated a surgical failure. If matters do not improve, such a patient rapidly becomes a chronic pain patient. Actually these are patients who are still suffering from their acute pathologic condition for a long time. Too often under these circumstances major therapeutic efforts on their behalf are directed toward assisting them to adapt to their various less than normal

situations in life. The physician should realize that there is probably an undiscovered acute pathologic lesion and that it requires assessment as though the patient were a new case. Account must be taken of the fact that the surgery that was performed may now cause confusing physical signs. This makes the discovery of the primary source of pain more difficult.

In one series six patients who had lumbar discs removed by uncomplicated surgical procedures, on recovering from the immediate effects of surgery, all complained of unremitting low back pain as it had existed before surgery. Because of this, none of them had been able to return to work. The lost work time was between 1 and 3 years in this small group of patients. On examination each one of them was found to be suffering from unrecognized and untreated acute, one-sided sacroiliac dysfunction on the same side as the leg pain. This was properly attended to, and immediate relief of pain was provided. The patients were all back to their normal employment within a month.

If one analyzes the various causes of pain in the musculoskeletal system, it is difficult to come up with any good reason why a prolapsed intervertebral disc should cause back pain. Such pain might arise from guarding muscle spasm, which should be readily relieved once the disc is removed and the direct results of surgery have healed. This is a logical place to take a critical look at the epidural space.

THE EPIDURAL SPACE

The boundaries of the epidural space are bony. Anteriorly there are vertebral bodies, laterally there are the pedicles, and posteriorly there are the laminae and their facets, which form intervertebral synovial joints. There are foramina through which the nerve roots pass as part of the peripheral nervous system. These lie superiorly in the foramina. The discs are more closely related to the interlaminar joints inferiorly, and swelling of them is more likely to press on the nerve roots than a bulging or prolapsed disc.

The normal contents of the epidural space are the spinal cord, the nerve roots, the conus medullaris, and the filum terminale. These are covered by their thecae. There are blood vessels, which may be in plexi. The theca contains the cerebrospinal fluid, whose normal presence maintains a constant pressure on all the structures within the space. The remaining space is filled with fat.

A large number of pathologic structures may invade the epidural space, which, being already full, cannot tolerate further intrusion. Intradural tumors, hematoma, or inflammatory conditions cause increased pressure within the epidural space. Extradural conditions will do the same thing. Among them are neuromas, epidural bleeding or hematoma, epidural abscesses, swelling of an interlaminar joint capsule, and hypertrophy of the ligamentum flavum. Calling everything that produces back pain with radiation a disc or a pinched nerve or discogenic disease has no true pathologic basis. Bone disease and bone tumors and posttraumatic callus may also directly invade the epidural space.

HEALING OR HEALED

Whatever the diagnostic entity is that is causing the pain, the clinician has to decide whether the pathologic state is in the healing phase or has already healed. This should be self-evident. Even so, there is no laboratory test, X-ray examination, or high-tech scan that can substitute for clinical judgment.

The importance of this decision has a bearing on the success or failure of treatment. If one decides to use modalities of treatment that are essentially designed to restore loss of function, the patient's condition will worsen if it has not healed. If the primary pathologic condition has healed and the patient continues on treatment designed to promote healing, then there will be no success in the restoration of function or strength. There is no place for manipulative therapy in the healing phase unless the diagnosis is mechanical (ie, joint dysfunction). Nevertheless, maintenance of joint play movements during the healing phase without any thought of restoring function during this period may be greatly appreciated when the patient reaches the healed or restorative phase of the disability.

The decision that a pathologic condition has healed and that the patient is ready to progress from the healing phase of a treatment program has to be based on clinical grounds. The clue to this change is found in the history that the patient gives. Usually during the healing phase the patient stiffens with rest. This stiffening may be resolved after an hour or two of activity, but it returns, often with increased pain, toward the end of the day. Improvement arrives when after rest there is no longer stiffness. The pain may be exacerbated once the patient starts activity. Too early a return to function can exacerbate symptoms again. Previously it has been remarked that with healing of a fracture the bone conduction of sound returns. This is an important clinical feature.

During the healing phase there are principles of treatment that must not be violated if morbid changes in the structures other than those that are affected in the primary pathologic condition are to be avoided. The principle that determines the formulation of a treatment program necessary for the healing process to occur is as follows: The structure in which the primary pathologic condition is located must be rested from function while all the other structures are maintained in as normal a physiologic state as possible. "Rest" does not mean "do not move." Such movement as may be used during the healing phase, however, must be passively administered by the therapist. This is a skillful procedure and is rarely performed properly by an assistant or an aide.

If a joint or muscle needs to be moved 10° and is only moved 5° during treatment, morbid changes occur in the structures not primarily involved. If such a joint or muscle is moved 15° when only 10° is indicated, then morbid changes occur in the structures not primarily involved. In the former case, this is the beginning of the morbid frozen joint. In the second case, this is the beginning of worsening of the primary pathologic condition. These threats of disaster should underscore the need for treatment by skilled professional persons. The right dosage of movement may change from day to day.

Manipulative treatment is contraindicated unless the diagnosis of the primary pathologic condition is mechanical. Exercise cannot restore intraarticular mechanical play within a joint. Therefore, the earlier mechanical treatment is used, the less therapy the patient requires on the road to normalcy.

In the healed phase, there is almost always a place for the restoration of normal intraarticular mechanics. This can only be achieved by a second person and not by self treatment.

The illogical habit of prescribing rest from function of a structure in the musculoskeletal system in which there is a pathologic change in an extremity and then to prescribe an exercise program for the same

pathologic change that may occur in the same structure in the back has to be abandoned. What is right in treating a structure in one part of the system is right in treating the same structure in any other part of the system. A muscle that may be the source of a pathologic change might be expected to respond to therapeutic exercises in a well-designed program.

Patients complain of symptoms in a topographic area of the musculoskeletal system. Patients may say that they have hurt their wrist, back, elbow, shoulder, foot, or ankle. That should be the last time that the physician should think in these terms. Chapter 4 indicates that each topographic area has to be broken down into its individual structures before a diagnosis can be made. One does not break one's wrist, one does not break one's back, one does not sprain one's ankle, and one cannot have bursitis or tenosynovitis where no anatomic bursae or tendon sheaths exist. Further, inflammation of bursae may herald disease, as may inflammation of the tendon sheath, unless there is a clear history of trauma at the onset of symptoms.

THE MANIPULATIVE LESION

Everything that humans make move has built-in mechanical play among the moving parts. It is not illogical to consider the human being the most perfect machine that was ever created. It is but a small step to believe that human synovial joints have this same characteristic. With experience, this can be shown to be true throughout the musculoskeletal system. These play movements in the human are logically designated the joint play movements. They are prerequisite to the performance of normal voluntary movements and function. Their loss impairs function and is associated with pain. The range of joint play movement is the same for any joint of the same kind in every normal person and should be considered the basis of normal kinesiology, that is to say normal living anatomy. The quantity of play may vary from joint to joint, but its quality is always the same. It is a sine qua non that, being a prerequisite of movement by the voluntary muscles, when joint play is impaired or lost it cannot be restored by any exercise program.

Loss of play in synovial joints is a mechanical diagnostic entity designated joint dysfunction, and this is a mechanical diagnosis of a cause of symptoms. It is common in any synovial joint anywhere in the system. To correct a mechanical fault it is logical to seek a mechanical form of treatment. This is joint manipulation.

Before orthodox medicine can accept a new diagnostic entity, it requires that there shall be present etiologic factors common to all the structures throughout the system. They are intrinsic trauma; immobilization, which must include disuse and aging; and residual pain, following some more serious pathologic condition. Without a doubt the best place to study this joint play–joint dysfunction–joint manipulation theory is in any orthopedic fracture clinic when immobilizing casts are being removed. Under these circumstances patients usually have an unaffected side in which normal play of the synovial joints can be demonstrated. On the affected side the loss of play may be clearly demonstrated by comparison with the normal.

Another prerequisite for the acceptance of joint play and its loss as being a cause of symptoms is the necessity to learn a system of physical examination that makes use of manipulative examining techniques. This is as difficult to learn from a book as it is for an aspiring artist to think that it is possible to learn painting from a paint by numbers kit. Yet, if the written word is followed faithfully, it obviously can be done.

RULES FOR JOINT PLAY EXAMINATION

For joint play movements to be examined, the patient must be recumbent. Only in this position does the examiner have perfect control of the examining movements that are being performed. The only exception to this is the examination of the joints of the fingers and the wrist. The position of examination is vital to the accumulation of precise data relating to joint movement. The techniques of eliciting joint play must be adhered to. It must be remembered that joint play movements are small in range. They are intraarticular and less than $\frac{1}{8}$ inch in any plane. Their performance requires accuracy and precision. To avoid patient resistance, one must stop each movement at the point of pain.

The rules are as follows:

1. The patient must be relaxed. Each aspect of the joint being examined must be supported and protected from unguarded painful movement that may otherwise occur in the course of the examination. Unguarded movements of painful joints produce pain that puts the supporting muscles into spasm and prevents a successful examination.

2. The examiner must be relaxed. At no time must the examining grip be painful to the patient. The grasp must be firm and protective but not restrictive: It must caress not constrict.

3. One joint must be examined at a time. For instance, when examining the wrist, the radiocarpal joint, the midcarpal joint, the ulnomeniscocarpal joint, and finally the inferior radioulnar joint are each examined in turn.

4. One movement at each joint is examined at a time.

5. In the performance of any one movement, one facet of the joint being examined is moved upon the other facet of the joint, which is stabilized. Thus there should always be one mobilizing force and one stabilizing force exerted when a joint is being examined.

6. The extent of normal joint play can usually be ascertained by examining

the same joint in the unaffected limb or the other side of the back.

7. No forceful movement must ever be used, and no abnormal movement must ever be used.
8. An examining movement must be stopped at any point at which pain is elicited.
9. In the presence of obvious clinical signs of inflammation or disease, no examining movements need to be or should be undertaken.

For technical reasons only should any of these rules be broken, and the reasons for breaking any rule must be clear. For instance, there is a long axis extension movement of joint play at every synovial joint in the body. When the wrist area is considered, it readily becomes obvious that one cannot test for this play movement at the radiocarpal joint without performing the same play movement at the midcarpal joint. Long axis extension of these two joints cannot be separated from long axis extension of the proximal radioulnar joint or from long axis extension of the glenohumeral joint unless the elbow is bent.

Other examples of the technical need to break rule 4 are found when considering the joints of the foot. The movement of rotational play of the bases of the metatarsal joints on the three cuneiform bones and the cuboid bones cannot be individualized. The anteroposterior glide movements of the three cuneiforms on the navicula, the talonavicular, or the calcaneocuboid joints cannot be individualized either.

The easiest joint in which to demonstrate play movements clinically, photographically, and radiologically is the second metacarpophalangeal joint. In Figures 5-48–5-50 these are shown. It should be noted that the image of the head of the metacarpal bone does not change in any of the pictures because it is stabilized. Its relationship to the base of the phalanx in each picture should be noted. It is then clear that voluntary movements are not being performed.

When voluntary movements are performed, both aspects of a joint move in relationship to each other throughout all ranges of movement. In play movements only the base of the phalanx is moved on the stabilized head of the metacarpal bone.

Play movements, other than long axis extension (distraction), are either tilting or shearing (gliding); that is, if one tilts when one should glide or glides when one should tilt, movement is achieved. The glide may be rotational as well as back and forth and from side to side.

Parenthetically, critics of this mechanical theory base their criticism on the fact that the ordinary tools of medical research cannot be used to demonstrate these facts. But joint play movements cannot be demonstrated on a cadaver, nor can they be produced by any action of voluntary muscle. All movements are lost in death.

Topographic reference to any musculoskeletal area must be abandoned. In the wrist, for instance, each joint is associated with a different functional movement:

- joint dysfunction at the radiocarpal joint is associated with loss of flexion of the wrist
- loss of joint play movements at the midcarpal joint is associated with loss of the voluntary movement of extension at the wrist
- joint dysfunction at the distal radioulnar joint is associated with loss of the voluntary movement of pronation
- joint dysfunction at the ulnotriquetral joint is associated with loss of the voluntary movement of supination

This is true in every topographic area of the musculoskeletal system. If more than one joint is involved in a topographic area, the cause of pain is not mechanical. In the back, if more than one side or one level is involved on manipulative examination, again the cause of pain is not mechanical.

It is often misleading to teach students by using acronyms. For instance, it is quite a common practice to limit the teaching of physical diagnosis of problems in the musculoskeletal system to two of these: ART and TART. The first T, if used, stands for tenderness; A stands for asymmetry; R stands for restriction of movement; and the last T stands for tissue tension change. All these things can be assessed on clinical examination, but they occur in every condition in the musculoskeletal system that presents the symptom of pain.

Thus assessment by the use of acronyms may tell where something is wrong but certainly not the nature of what is wrong. Acronyms are, therefore, of little use in the differential diagnostic field. The basis of medicine is correct diagnosis, accurate prognosis, and treatment that has a predictable result.

There are five generic categories of diagnosable conditions that produce pain in the musculoskeletal system. This need not necessarily be from the system itself. It is difficult in these days of high-tech diagnostic medicine and the practice of defensive medicine to persuade audiences that in facing the problems of the musculoskeletal system we remain in a clinical field. One receives little support in diagnostic efforts from any of the ancillary tests available to those who practice in almost any other field of medicine. For diagnosis we must rely on clinical examination: listening, feeling, and thinking. Perhaps the most important of these is listening. A simple example, close to the subject we are discussing, is when a patient relates that he or she did something to a knee and it locked. Few physicians would hesitate to do something to unlock that knee manipulatively. When a child suddenly develops a paralyzing pain in the elbow because he or she was pulled by the arm, it would be a rare physician who failed to recognize that the child is suffering from a pulled elbow. As soon as possible the physician would reduce the subluxation, which is really joint dysfunction, manipulatively. Nevertheless, few physicians would try to unlock any part of the back

manipulatively because the back remains mysterious. It has yet to be recognized as just a part of the musculoskeletal system. The teaching is that most theories regarding back pain have been disproved, which is reason enough not to manipulate patients with back pain. It is difficult to overcome dogma by logic or common sense, but the following paragraphs attempt to do just that. Tables 3-1 and 3-2 at the end of this chapter illustrate how to differentiate by clinical means the probable causes of symptoms, which allows the cause to be treated rather than any one symptom.

Assuming that there is a diagnosable condition that responds to manipulative therapy and that we call synovial joint dysfunction, it must be possible to differentiate symptoms and signs of this condition from the symptoms and signs arising from other pathologic conditions. These include pathologic conditions that involve synovial joints and pathologic conditions that attack the synovial capsule and ligaments and occur in muscles, menisci, and intervertebral discs. These also occur in bursae, in neoplastic conditions, in bone and joint diseases, and as a result of congenital anomalies. Moreover, it must be possible to differentiate all these musculoskeletal causes of pain from symptoms referred to the system from systemic and organ disease.

Clues are to be found in our observations of pain, its onset, its nature, and its localization. Clinical examination must look for changes in skin temperature and color; movement restrictions require interpretation. Joint swelling must be observed, and swelling must be differentiated on the basis of that which occurs within the joint capsule and that which occurs outside it.

Excess intraarticular fluid may be due to too much synovial fluid. This is found after trauma and in disease processes. It may be due to blood after trauma, or it may be due to blood diseases such as hemophilia. Tumors such as pigmented villonodular synovitis, which may be locally invasive but not malignant, cause spontaneous bleeding. Excess fluid may be due to other tumors of a malignant nature. It may be due to pus. These things can be recognized generically by clinical means: The swelling of excess synovial fluid is usually quite large and takes some time to develop because the fluid is normal to the joint; it does not set up inflammatory changes, and therefore the joint is warm but not hot. When first seen the joint is often large. Because there is no inflammation, there is no acute pain but rather a stiffness and aching. There may be no appreciable muscle atrophy.

Compare this with blood in a joint. Blood is foreign to the joint and sets up an acute inflammatory reaction. This is hot and painful. When first seen the swelling may be quite small because of the inherent clotting mechanism. If it is not attended to, excess synovial fluid is added to the blood, and the size of the joint may be increased. This could be misleading. The onset of symptoms is sudden, but there is no early evidence of muscle atrophy.

If the fluid is due to pus or its precursor, the onset of joint symptoms occurs during a primary infectious condition, and the patient may have been sick for 10 days or more before the joint manifestations occur. This is particularly true in children. Acute hematogenous synovitis is an urgent surgical condition. It is a cause of pseudoparesis in children.

There are two causes of infected joints that have unusual characteristics. The first is the tubercular joint, in which the swelling may be small but the accompanying muscle atrophy seems to be excessive for the joint disability. The second is the gonococcal joint, which is not especially swollen and in which the muscle is not notably atrophied. Nevertheless, the pain is sufficiently severe that the patient withdraws as the physician approaches to examine it. Pus and blood have lysins in them that destroy hyaline cartilage. If these fluids are not removed, severe destructive

degenerative changes occur within the joint. There is one kind of synovial joint change that occurs when the cause is syphilis, diabetes, or spinal cord injuries. This is the Charcot joint. When established, it is painless. At the onset of joint involvement, however, there may be considerable pain that is diagnostically overlooked because of later painlessness. There is one other cause of painful joint swelling, and this may be called a reactive synovitis. It occurs as a manifestation, for instance, of serum sickness and as a response in patients with some allergic problems.

Joint dysfunction, which is the manipulatable lesion, does not manifest any evidence of external trauma or inflammation, and this is a clear differentiation from the many causes that have been discussed. There are three characteristic clinical signs that preclude making a mechanical diagnosis. First, if on palpation of a joint it is possible to feel the joint capsule, the cause of symptoms is not mechanical. Second, one cannot palpate fluid in a normal joint. The presence of fluid of any kind that is palpable in a joint capsule precludes making a mechanical diagnosis. Third is an observation that may be the most important of all. Normal ligaments are never tender on palpation. If there is tenderness that appears to be arising from a ligament, and if there is no reason by history to suppose that there could have been ligament injury at the onset of pain, then there is something wrong with the joint that the ligament supports. In the back, there is something wrong with the junction that the ligament supports, whatever the cause.

The importance of knowing the anatomic locale of the ligaments of the synovial joints is made clear by the following example. Ankle pain may be arising from one of two joints: the mortise joint or the subtalar joint. Which of these is the source of pain can most accurately be decided by palpation through the sinus tarsi. The examining finger increases pressure at the base of this anatomic structure, and there lies the only palpable ligament specific to the subtalar joint. Tenderness elicited by this simple clinical examining procedure precludes the diagnosis of anything being wrong with the mortise joint.

SIGNIFICANT DIAGNOSTIC POINTS IN HISTORY TAKING

Returning for a moment to the importance of listening, the history of ankle pain is characteristic for each joint at the ankle. If the mortise joint is the source of symptoms, the patient complains of the pain worsening when walking uphill or upstairs. If the subtalar joint is the source of pain, then it is worse when walking downhill or downstairs. The above are all objective clinical observations that any medical student should be expected to note and to use in a diagnostic exercise. The observations that follow require listening and some interpretive experience. They concern history taking, the nature of the symptom of pain, and the effects of rest and activity on it.

The pain of joint dysfunction commonly comes on suddenly and during movement, with or without an unexpected movement being superimposed. There are three etiologic factors that are prerequisites for making the diagnosis of joint dysfunction: intrinsic trauma; immobilization, which includes disuse and aging; and residual pain after healing of a more serious pathologic condition. The onset of pain from joint dysfunction arising from these last two etiologic factors may be insidious and at rest. Listening to the historical sequence of events should readily clarify the situation.

The onset of muscle pain from muscle fiber tears and tendon tears is usually sudden and occurs during movement. Yet the onset of pain from multiple or repetitive microtrauma to muscles and their tendons may be insidious and at rest. A rotator cuff tear in patients older than 50 years of age may be spontaneous and intrinsic. In such cases the history of the onset of shoulder pain may be confusing. Capsular and ligament pain, unless arising from tears or sprains, is usually insidious in onset and is not associated with any remembered trauma.

The onset of pain from a prolapsed disc is usually sudden and during movement. There is often a history of an earlier predisposing back injury. In contrast, the onset of pain from local disease in a skeletal structure is usually insidious. Night pain is suggestive of bone tumor. The onset of pain in the musculoskeletal system arising from systemic disease is also insidious and while the patient is resting.

Effect of Rest on Pain

The effects of rest and activity on pain are often characteristic of a diagnostic entity. Rest relieves the pain of joint dysfunction and, in the back, of disc prolapse. In all the other conditions that we are discussing (except for systemic disease, in which rest has no specific effect on pain), stiffening occurs with rest, and sometimes pain may be worsened by rest.

Effect of Activity on Pain

Activity, and often one movement more than another, reproduces the pain of joint dysfunction and, in the back, of disc prolapse. Activity initially relieves the pain of local disease and of the other causes of musculoskeletal pain except systemic disease, but continued activity reproduces and aggravates the pain. Thus from history taking alone one can begin to develop a diagnostic suspicion as to the cause of musculoskeletal pain.

SIMPLE DIAGNOSTIC CLUES FROM OBSERVATION

Patient's Localization of Pain

The patient with joint dysfunction causing symptoms can usually localize the source by pointing with a finger. This is true for pain in the extremities and the back. If the source of pain in the back is a disc prolapse, the patient localizes the level quite well. Pain from bone or joint disease is usually not well localized. When pain arises from dysfunction, it is unilateral. Pain from disease obviously involves more than one joint. In the back the signs are bilateral and at one or more levels.

Patients are unable to localize the source of muscle pain in the back, but in the extremities localization is usually good. An exception is when the cause of pain is an irritable trigger point. In such a case the patient has no idea of the locality of the source of the pain and can only indicate a pattern of pain, usually far removed from the source. Pain may be referred from a joint, and yet its localization is not well demonstrated. The patient sometimes complains of knee joint pain and a limp when the pathologic condition giving rise to the pain is really arising from the hip joint.

Earlier in this book attention was drawn to the diagnostic problem of joint pain manifesting itself as visceral pain. Also, visceral pathology gives rise to what would appear to be joint pain. To help differentiate these two things, it is important to note whether or not there are architectural changes in any of the skeletal structures. This is especially true in the back, where there will be abnormal segmental curves to the right or left, segmental flattening of the normal lordotic curve, or a locally increased kyphosis. Obviously, segmental changes within the spinal curves do not initially occur as the result of visceral or systemic disorders unless there is bone involvement because of the primary disease metastasizing from

it. Sacral pain is usually referred to the sacrum from some organic cause within the pelvis unless there is a clear history of direct trauma to it. A hairline fracture of the sacrum after direct trauma is difficult to diagnose and is resistant to treatment.

Architectural Changes in Spinal Curves

In the absence of preexisting disease or congenital anomaly, no one can alter the levelness of the iliac crests or change any part of a spinal curve segmentally without alteration of stance. The cause of the pain is likely to be joint dysfunction in the sacroiliac joint, the facet joint of the lumbosacral junction, or the fourth lumbar junction on the side of the pain.

If the patient indicates that the pain is on the side of the lowered iliac crest and of the concavity of the sciatic scoliosis, a disc prolapse between the fourth and fifth lumbar vertebrae or at the lumbosacral junction should be suspected. Sometimes sciatic scoliosis changes from side to side during the clinical examination. In such a case a disc prolapse may be the cause. Local spinal disease produces segmental architectural changes, but the changes are likely to be flattening of a curve or the presence of a gibbous deformity.

Inferences To Be Drawn from Impaired Movement

All musculoskeletal conditions in which pain is a feature are associated with impaired or lost movement so long as ligamentous integrity is maintained. A torn ligament is associated with excess movement, which may be masked by muscle spasm. Musculoskeletal pain associated with systemic disease does not impair movement.

Impairment of forward bending is characteristic of all low back problems but in itself is of no clinical significance except that it tells the examiner that something is wrong and provides a baseline from which to observe objectively improvement or deterioration. The manner of return to upright from the stooped position is clinically significant. However limited forward bending may be, the patient with joint dysfunction or a disc prolapse recovers the upright position normally. In contrast, a patient with some more serious pathologic condition and especially with local spinal disease recovers the upright position tortuously and slowly.

Significance of Vertebral Percussion

The property of long bone to conduct sound has already been described. Percussion also produces pain at the site of a fracture. This is called Stimson's sign. Percussion of bone in which there is a pathologic condition also produces a sickening pain at the pathologic site. There is an interesting phenomenon in which bone pain is associated with true muscle trigger points. For instance, pain on percussion of the lateral condyle of the humerus is associated with a trigger point in the extensor carpi radialis. Often this bone pain is the first physical sign to disappear when that trigger point is recognized as the source of pain and is properly treated. A trigger point in the masseter muscle gives rise to lower jaw pain, which the patient describes as severe toothache.

Percussion over individual vertebra produces pain when the source of symptoms is in the bone or in the junction below it. If the source is an intervertebral disc, the jarring of the vertebra by percussion often aggravates or reproduces the radiated pain. If the source is joint dysfunction, percussion of the vertebra produces a short, sharp pain. In the presence of bone or joint disease or some inflammatory epidural lesion, the pain is deep, dull, and aching. It may be a sickening, throbbing pain.

The reaction of a patient to vertebral percussion and the way in which a patient recovers the upright position from the forward bending position are perhaps the two most characteristic features of a back examination. These differentiate pain from mechanical joint dysfunction and serious vertebral disease.

Skin Rolling and Vertebral Springing Tests

Normally the skin rolls over the back freely and painlessly. When a patient with back pain is subjected to skin rolling over the spine, the examiner may feel a tissue texture change in the form of tightness at any level of pathologic change.

If skin rolling is then performed paravertebrally, the examiner feels a similar tightness at the same level on the side of the pain and less tightness, if any, on the opposite side. Then the cause of pain is most likely to be mechanical. If the paravertebral tightness is bilateral, the diagnosis of a mechanical cause of symptoms is precluded. At the areas where tightness is felt, the patient experiences pain that may be acute.

Skin rolling is useful in the extremities, but the cause of changes is less easily interpreted. In the back a positive skin rolling test indicates the level of where something is wrong. Also, if the test is positive unilaterally and at one level, then the source is likely to be a facet joint with a mechanical problem, a prolapsed disc, or a local muscle tear. If the physical signs are bilateral or multilevel, then some more serious pathologic condition must be contemplated.

Neurologic Signs

In dealing with the back there is an additional clinical test which confirms the intervertebral level at which pathologic change should be sought.

Although joint dysfunction and muscle trigger points give rise to referred pain, they do not produce radiating pain. There are not any neurologic signs that are characteristic of either of these conditions. A prolapsed disc is usually associated with radiating pain and mixed (motor and sensory) neurologic signs. Local spine disease is characterized early by changing neurologic signs that require repeated examinations to detect. Interspinous ligament tenderness is a good indication of the level of spine pathology but gives no clue as to its nature. After surgical procedures, nerve elements may be entrapped in scar tissue, signs of which may confuse the assessment of postoperative pain.

All these clinical observations are objective. The clinical picture of joint dysfunction is made up of clear etiologic factors, symptoms, and objective clinical signs. When the diagnosis is clear, relief by manipulative therapy is predictable.

Radiologic and Laboratory Observations

There are no characteristic radiologic changes associated with joint dysfunction. In the early stage of musculoskeletal diseases, X-ray examinations are of little if any diagnostic help. The laboratory may be of no assistance either. Special X-ray techniques may be helpful, but they are expensive and need not be used unless there is good reason. Myelograms, discograms, venograms, epidurograms, tomograms, cineradiograms, bone scans, computed tomograms, and magnetic resonance images may all have their place, but they should not be used until a presumptive clinical diagnosis has been reached. The same pertains to the use of electromyography and thermography, both of which can now be relegated to research projects.

Assuming that the history and examination have ruled out neurologic disease as the cause of symptoms, the following are important points. A raised protein level in the cerebrospinal fluid must be indicative of some pathology that is probably treatable. A raised erythrocyte sedimentation rate in the absence of other changes in laboratory tests is suggestive of malignancy. Characteristic changes in the values of calcium, phosphorus, and alkaline phosphatase are diagnostically important.

An unusual clinical test in the United States is an epidural injection of 2% saline. It is a useful diagnostic test to detect encroachment of the epidural space. It is also a therapeutic tool to relieve the pain of nerve root edema and epidural adhesions. The sacrococcygeal hiatus is used for introduction of the saline. Local and radiating pain is experienced by the patient when the injected fluid reaches the level of an epidural obstruction. Relief of pain is experienced if the pain symptom is caused by nerve root edema or epidural adhesions around a nerve root.

Other Clinical Observations

There are three simple observations that aid in arriving at a differential diagnosis of the cause of pain in the musculoskeletal system. The presence of intraarticular swelling has been commented on, and the examination of the involved part of the system for increased warmth and heat has been touched upon.

Skin discoloration may occur. Bruising is commonly observed in the extremities and is evidence of bleeding. In the back, similar injuries that cause bleeding in the extremities must also cause bleeding in the back. Because the back is so thick and because the lumbodorsal fascia is so protective, there is no way for blood to rise to the surface and become apparent as skin discoloration. If the bleeding is life threatening it must first be corrected, before other musculoskeletal injuries are considered in detail. Perhaps it is unnecessary to remind the reader that there is a similarity between occult bleeding in the back and intracranial, intrathoracic, and intraabdominal bleeding. Evidence of these never reaches the surface of the body. Nevertheless, it is illogical to assume that bleeding does not happen just because one cannot visualize it from the surface of the body. If bleeding is ignored during the healing phase of structural damage, organization of the blood is followed by the formation of fibrous tissue. Scarring makes the restoration phase of treatment of such injuries more difficult.

SUMMARY

Except as a result of gross trauma, nothing ever happens to the back or to any other topographic area in the musculoskeletal system. Pathologic changes occur at the junctions in the back, and that should give one pause in talking about or treating the back for pain.

Physical examination of any part of the musculoskeletal system never should involve patient activity, if only because loss of function is one of the chief complaints that brings the patient to the physician. The action of the muscles of the back is all or none. Problems at any intervertebral junction are masked by attempted voluntary movement. Intervertebral movements are joint play movements, and their presence or loss can only be detected by examining manipulative techniques. It is important to remember that normal joint play movements are prerequisites to efficient, pain-free voluntary movements. This is a principle of mechanics. Simple loss of joint play after intrinsic trauma is a common, diagnosable cause of synovial joint pain wherever there are synovial joints in the system.

The only treatment that relieves the pain of joint dysfunction is therapeutic manipulation that concerns itself only with restoring lost movements of play. The only indication for the use of joint manipulation is to relieve this diagnostic cause of pain, not the pain itself. In the absence of this diagnosis, joint manipulation as a therapy is contraindicated.

Tables 3-1, 3-2, and 3-3 are summaries of what this chapter is all about. The column titled joint dysfunction in all three tables shows the positive things that are relatively simple to elicit and interpret once they are properly learned. Unless most of the items in this column are present, there is no indication for the use of joint manipulation as a primary treatment.

One must remember that there are two other etiologic factors besides intrinsic trauma that give rise to joint dysfunction. The onset of pain may be insidious rather than during movement. In those cases manipulative therapy may have to be delayed. Pain clinic personnel should have a clear understanding of the potential use of manipulative therapy when supposedly dealing with chronic pain problems arising from the musculoskeletal system. Patients do not have to learn to adapt to pain caused by joint dysfunction. They predictably can be cured.

Just as there is more than one etiologic factor to be taken into account before making the diagnosis of joint dysfunction, so there are two etiologic factors to be considered before making a diagnosis of some muscle pathology. The onset of pain because of tears and ruptures occurs suddenly and during movement. In some industrial occupations, however, cumulative multiple microtrauma may be associated with work, and the onset of pain may be insidious.

When mobility is considered in the clinical examination, the examiner should remember to measure the distance between the posterior and superior iliac spines with the patient sitting and later when prone. Absence of movement between these bones with change of posture is pathognomonic of sacroiliac joint disease. If this happens to be ankylosing spondylitis, then a

Table 3-1 Highlights of Pain by History

Lesion Characteristics	Trauma				Disease		
	Joint Dysfunction	Muscle Pathology	Disc Prolapse		Local Disease	Systemic Disease	
Onset	Etiology: intrinsic trauma—sudden during movement Etiology: immobilization and after healing of more serious pathology—insidious at rest	Tears: sudden during movement Multiple microtrauma: insidious at rest	Sudden during movement		Insidious at rest	Insidious at rest	
Effect of rest	Relieves pain	Stiffness with/without relief of pain	Relieves pain		Stiffness and pain may increase	No effect	
Effect of activity	Aggravates, but not with all movements	Aggravates, especially on stretching of muscle	Aggravates, especially radiating pain		Initial relief followed by aggravation All movements Night pain with bone tumor	Fatigues easily	

Table 3-2 Ancillary Means of Diagnosis

Lesion Characteristics	Trauma			Disease	
	Joint Dysfunction	Muscle Pathology	Disc Prolapse	Local Disease	Systemic Disease
Localization of pain by pointing	Accurate: most often unilateral	Indefinite but usually one sided	Accurate: usually unilateral	Accurate: central and bilateral	Indefinite
Architectural	Low back: Sciatic scoliosis convex on side of pain; Iliac crest raised on side of pain; Neck: usually flattening; Chest: segmental flattening	No architectural change	Low back: Sciatic scoliosis concave on side of pain; Iliac crest low on side of pain; Sciatic scoliosis may change from side to side; No characteristic change in neck or chest	Segmental flattening or gibbus contour	No architectural change
Mobility*	Low back: Localized—loss of forward bending; Recovery normal; Impaired upright rotation in ipsilateral direction of sacroiliac joint. Thoracic spine: Localized—loss of forward bending; Recovery normal; Impaired rotation in one direction. Cervical spine: Loss of rotation in one direction and side bending on the other	Poorly localized loss; Recovery may be tortuous	Low back: Localized loss—recovery normal. Cervical spine: Side bending with/without rotation to side of arm pain restricted by radiating pain	Localized loss (or excess movement above level of involvement); Recovery tortuous	Possible generalized loss; Recovery may be tortuous; No change in distance between posterior-superior iliac spines with change of posture equals sacroiliac joint disease

	Column A	Column B	Column C	Column D	Column E
Vertebral percussion	Sharp pain at involved junction	No pain	Sharp pain with reproduction of radiating pain	Deep, throbbing, aching pain	No characteristic reaction
Skin rolling†	Tight and tender over vertebra above involved junction and worse on side of pain (unilateral)	No abnormality over vertebra. Tight and tender over involved area of muscle	Tight and tender over vertebra above involved junction. Unilateral tenderness on side of radiating pain	Tight and tender over involved vertebra and junction. Bilateral paravertebral involvement	Tight and tender either all over or scattered all over back
Vertebral springing‡	One-level pain	No pain	One-level pain	One or more levels of pain	None
Neurologic signs	None	None	Mixed	Changing early	None unless disease is neurologic
General observations	Patient lies still. No signs of systemic disease. No fever	Patient varies position. No signs of systemic disease. No fever	Patient lies still. Not ill and no fever unless disc infection or epidural abscess present	Patient lies still. Possible signs of systemic disease and fever may occur	Patient restless. May sit up or roll up. Signs of systemic disease and fever common

*When testing mobility measure the distance between the posterior-superior iliac spines with the patient sitting and then prone. Absence of movement is pathognomonic of sacroiliac disease. Also measure the respiratory excursion of the chest: It is diminished with ankylosing spondylitis.

†Skin rolling over the iliotibial bands is a good way of detecting tenderness in a tight band. Tight and tender iliotibial bands cause recurrent sacroiliac joint pain when unilateral and lumbosacral junction pain when bilateral.

‡When springing a vertebra elicits pain, that pain is coming either from the vertebra being sprung or the junction below it.

Table 3-3 X-ray and Laboratory Findings

Lesion Characteristics	Trauma			Disease	
	Joint Dysfunction	Muscle Pathology	Disc Prolapse	Local Disease	Systemic Disease
Characteristic X-ray findings	None	None	None except with special techniques	None early	None early; then osteoporosis
				Bone scan or tomogram may show changes earlier than routine radiographs	Simple osteoporosis never affects skull or lamina dura
Laboratory findings	None	None	Cerebrospinal fluid protein level raised	Blood count changes	Blood count changes
				Increased erythrocyte sedimentation rate	Increased erythrocyte sedimentation rate
				Possible changes in chemistries	Altered blood chemistries
				Protein in urine @ 60°	

diminished respiratory excursion is likely also.

A part of the low back examination is to skin roll over the iliotibial bands. If there is tightness and tenderness on performing this test, treatment to overcome these two things should be part of the overall therapeutic program. Unilateral tightness and tenderness tend to cause recurrence of symptoms because of recurrent sacroiliac dysfunction; bilateral tightness and tenderness cause recurrence of dysfunction symptoms at the lumbosacral junction.

The following items also are important:

1. When a patient complains of back pain and abdominal pain, look for the source in the abdomen if the pains are at the same level.

2. When a patient complains of back pain and abdominal pain and if the abdominal pain is at a lower level than the back pain, look for the source in the back.

3. Sacral pain is always a symptom of visceral pain unless there is a clear history of direct trauma to the sacrum.

4. In the back pain patient whose symptoms are of obscure origin, remember to do a rectal examination and a pelvic examination if appropriate.

5. Always remember to use a clinical thermometer when faced with a patient with musculoskeletal pain.

6. The importance of feeling the pulses of all four extremities in patients with back and extremity pain cannot be too highly stressed. These may be the clue to the diagnosis of the thoracic outlet syndrome, aneurysms, coarctation of the aorta, and Leriche's syndrome (a saddle thrombus at the bifurcation of the aorta).

chapter 4

Clinical Examination

HISTORY TAKING

To some readers it may seem odd that history taking is relegated to a relatively late chapter when it should already be clear from the beginning that the author follows the teaching of Sir William Osler, which starts with the exhortation to his students to listen to the patient.

In Chapter 3 differential diagnosis is touched upon, and Tables 3-1, 3-2, and 3-3 attempt to differentiate the various syndromes that must be compared with each other by the use of diagnostic guidelines. Reference to Table 3-1 indicates how to identify the loss of mechanical joint play, which constitutes the diagnosis of mechanical joint dysfunction. Primary joint dysfunction is the manipulable lesion. Its elective and predictably effective treatment is joint manipulation.

This is the only pathologic condition that should be manipulated in the healing phase. If one accepts this, then conditions that make up the syndromes described in columns 2 to 5 in the tables are contraindications for the use of manipulative therapy during the healing phase, whether the symptoms are arising from changes in structures within the system or whether the symptoms are referred to the system from some other system. In the healed phase of any pathologic condition that falls in columns 2 to 5, there is seldom a patient who would not benefit from joint manipulation of some joints somewhere in the system, whatever other modalities may be prescribed.

In considering the problems of the musculoskeletal system, it is necessary first to establish the system before honing in on an approach to that system in health and in sickness. Once the system is established, then the student can return to the more usual approach in physical examination.

Causes of Musculoskeletal Pain

All causes of pain appreciated by a patient as being of the musculoskeletal system produce the same symptoms and signs as if the pain were arising within the system. These are tenderness, asymmetry, restriction of movement, and tissue texture changes. From these things alone, all that we know is that there is something wrong in the musculoskeletal system. Pain is not a diagnosis, however; it is merely a symptom.

Emphasis is placed on two causes of pain that are frequently overlooked and yet are predictably diagnosable once their existence is acknowledged: Travell's trigger points (Chapter 6) and mechanical joint dysfunction (Chapter 3). Just as there are many clues in a patient's history of muscle and joint pain that may point to the diagnosis of joint disease, so also are there clues available from a patient's history that strongly suggest the diagnosis of these two relatively unrecognized conditions. There is little new, therefore, in the following paragraphs of history taking from a patient complaining of musculoskeletal symptoms (especially pain), but some of the interpretation of the various points in the history may be found to have a new significance.

Etiologic Factors Predisposing to Joint Dysfunction

Primary joint dysfunction commonly results from the imposition of some unguarded movement at a joint that at the time is actively going through a normal functional movement. It may also commonly follow some definite traumatic episode of a minor nature involving the joint, the immediate effects of which are usually diagnosed as sprains or strains. In the former case, the trauma to the joint is intrinsic, whereas in the latter case it is extrinsic. The recognition that a joint can be injured from an intrinsic cause is essential to the appreciation of the condition of joint dysfunction.

Joint dysfunction is perhaps the commonest cause of residual symptoms after severe bone and joint injury and after almost every joint disease when the primary pathologic condition has been eradicated, has healed, or is quiescent. Joint dysfunction commonly occurs in joints that have been immobilized in the treatment of fractures, even though there may be no particular reason to believe that the joints themselves were involved in the traumatic incident that caused the fractures. It may also follow immobilization occasioned either by severe soft tissue injury around the joint or by treatment after surgery. It is also the commonest cause of residual symptoms after any inflammatory condition of a joint or after the resolution of any systemic disease that involves joint structures. It may or may not be associated with the presence of intraarticular adhesions. The reader should refer to Tables 3-1, 3-2, and 3-3, which summarize the difference in historical features for each generic category of the causes of pain anywhere in the system.

Etiologic Factors Predisposing to Trigger Points

Because myofascial trigger points as described by Travell occur in the same location in any given muscle in anyone, one has to make the assumption that trigger points are latent in muscle and only give rise to symptoms when they are irritated by some primary cause. This means that an irritable trigger point initially is a secondary phenomenon and that pain from it is masked by the primary pain from the primary pathologic condition. Most frequently, when the primary cause of pain is resolved, any trigger point pain may well be resolved also. Muscles learn bad habits quickly and unlearn them slowly if at all, however, and then they become a primary source of pain that requires diagnosis and treatment.

For instance, the somatic component of the visceral pain from coronary artery thrombosis may persist long after a patient has recovered from the precipitating heart attack. This pseudoangina should not be looked upon as evidence that the patient is becoming or has become a cardiac invalid. The pain in such an instance may well be coming from an irritable trigger point that was set off by the cardiac condition but is not a true part of it. Another example of this phenomenon would be residual pain after surgical removal of a fourth lumbar disc with the patient complaining of persistent leg pain in spite of the fact that the primary cause of it has been properly removed. A trigger point in the gluteus minimus exhibits a pattern of referred pain that mimics the radiating pain caused by the prolapsed disc. Thus the etiologic factors that give rise to irritational trigger points may arise from any local injury sustained by any part of the musculoskeletal system or because of pain referred to the musculoskeletal system from any other cause of systemic disease or visceral pathology. It is interesting that the referred pain from an irritable trigger point, when it is recognized, responds just as well whether the pain is of recent origin or whether the patient has suffered from it for a long time.

One etiologic factor is likely to be overlooked because it is very common after surgery, and every surgeon has a different explanation for this kind of pain. In amputees, neuroma pain often is due to pain referred from a trigger point in one of the muscles traumatized by the surgery.

Whenever the chest is opened by a thoracic or cardiac surgeon, the postoperative pain is often caused either by joint dysfunction of the thoracic facet joints or the costovertebral joints or by intercostal or chest wall muscle trigger points that have become irritable because of the surgical procedure or because of pain referred from the dysfunctional joints (or both).

PRESENT COMPLAINT

Onset of Symptoms

The history of the onset of the joint symptoms may suggest a diagnosis. The onset of symptoms is either sudden or insidious. If the onset is sudden and fol-

lows a remembered traumatic episode but is not accompanied by associated joint swelling, joint dysfunction is a likely diagnosis. If the onset is sudden and the pain is accompanied by swelling of the joint, it is unlikely that joint dysfunction is the primary cause of the patient's symptoms; it is more probable that the symptoms are due to some pathologic change in one or more of the other six anatomic structures that make up the joint. If the onset of symptoms is sudden, following, for instance, the removal of some supporting device that has been worn for any length of time and coinciding with the resumption of activity, then it is most likely that the cause of pain is joint dysfunction.

If the onset of symptoms is insidious, joint dysfunction is a most unlikely diagnosis. It should be remembered, however, that intrinsic trauma to a joint may occur during sleep without wakening the patient and that the patient may only notice the discomfort or pain on waking. In such cases, when trauma is not recalled and the onset is considered insidious, the history must not be allowed to confuse the issue.

If more than one joint is involved and if the onset of pain occurred at about the same time, joint dysfunction can be the cause only if the involved joints have been immobilized as part of treatment (eg, after multiple fractures, burns, or a single fracture in which the immobilizing cast extends over more than one joint) or if there is a clear history of a traumatic episode that definitely involves all the joints in which there is pain.

Nature of Joint Pain

The pain of joint dysfunction tends to be sharp and occurs, often only intermittently, when the joint is in function, the same movement always causing recurrence of the pain. It is almost always relieved by rest. When joint dysfunction causes residual symptoms after a primary joint disease or injury has been eradicated or becomes quiescent, the history of the nature of the pain changes. It is this change in the nature of the pain that gives the clue that the residual symptoms in the joint are probably arising from joint dysfunction. During the phase of active disease, for example, the patient finds that the pain is possibly worse after rest and that the joint stiffens with rest, whereas with joint dysfunction the patient finds that the pain is improved by rest and is disturbing only when the joint is used.

Joint pain that is disturbing to the patient on waking in the morning, is less severe after he or she limbers up with perhaps an hour or more of activity, and then worsens again toward the end of the day is seldom due to joint dysfunction. Night pain that wakens the patient is often due to bone disease or neoplasm.

The pain of joint disease is most often deep, aching, and throbbing; it may be lessened by pressure, just as the ache from an infected tooth may be somewhat relieved by pressing on it. This type of pain may be constant or occur in waves or spasms, and it may be sharp or dull. The pain of joint dysfunction is invariably sharp; it usually ceases immediately when the stressful action that produces it ceases; it is invariably relieved or at least markedly improved by rest and aggravated by activity. Thus the patient's answers to questions as to what aggravates and what improves the pain may be significant.

Localization of Pain

The localization of the pain by the patient is sometimes most helpful in giving a clue to a correct diagnosis, for often patients are able to indicate clearly in which component of the joint the pain seems to be situated when the pathologic condition causing the pain is not joint dysfunction. In the areas of the limbs where there are multiple joints, the localization of the pain by the patient will often draw attention to the specific joint from which the pain is arising and in which dysfunction may be present.

Loss of Movement and Pain

In the joints of the limbs, each movement in the range of joint play is always associated with the ability to perform some particular voluntary motion. For instance, extension at the wrist for the most part occurs at the midcarpal joint. If a patient is unable to extend the wrist, this fact should draw attention to the movements of joint play upon which the voluntary movement of extension depends, namely those that are associated with the midcarpal joint. In the same region, inability of the patient to perform supination of the forearm after, for example, a Colles' fracture should draw attention to the joint play movements associated with the ulnomeniscotriquetral joint. The inferior radioulnar joint is associated with pronation of the forearm and hand.

PAST HISTORY

The past history of a patient complaining of joint pain must be inquired into, for therein may lie the clue to the true nature of the pathologic cause of the pain. A past history of heart disease in childhood, chorea, or St Vitus' dance suggests that the cause of pain may be acute rheumatic fever. Migraine or allergic conditions such as asthma or hay fever suggest a diagnosis of nonspecific intermittent hydrarthrosis. A chronic cough, loss of weight, unexplained pyrexia, undue sweating, and the drinking of raw milk in the past suggest that the underlying cause of the joint symptoms may be tuberculosis or brucellosis, whereas fleeting pains in the small joints of the extremities are suggestive of rheumatoid arthritis. Joint pain after dietary extravagance may suggest gout, and the history of a recent injection of antitoxin or the administration of a new drug might suggest an allergic basis for the joint symptoms. Recent venereal disease may mean gonococcal arthritis, and syphilis may be manifested by either synovial joint or bone involvement. The history of recent intraarticular injections of medication or of joint aspiration may suggest the onset of pyarthrosis. In joints in which there are intraarticular fibrocartilages (menisci), a past history of locking of the joint with pain strongly suggests meniscal injury.

The past history may reveal illness while traveling abroad, and it should be remembered that hydatid disease, amebiasis, fungal infections, and some rare tropical diseases may manifest themselves as joint pain in their chronic course. Acquired immunodeficiency syndrome (AIDS) and Lyme disease must be added to the long list of different diagnoses of joint pain.

FAMILY HISTORY

The patient's family history should not be forgotten, for there is a tendency for rheumatic diseases to be familial. This work, however, is not concerned with the more esoteric causes of joint pain such as ochronosis and hemophilia, from which the differentiation of joint dysfunction should present no problem.

SYSTEM REVIEW

A complete review of a patient's visceral systems should be undertaken because joint pain may be the presenting feature of systemic disease such as lupus erythematosus, scleroderma, dermatomyositis, Reiter's disease, erythema nodosum, and polyarteritis nodosa. Symptoms of joint pain may rarely be associated with and draw attention to acromegaly, pulmonary disease, kidney disease, and Henoch's purpura and other hemorrhagic dyscrasias. Arthralgia may also be associated with ulcerative colitis.

Pain in a joint may be referred from disease of distant viscera, which can be diagnosed only by careful system review. Classic examples of this include a wide variety of conditions often causing referred pain in a shoulder joint. A few of these are coronary artery disease, pericarditis, lesions in other parts of the mediastinum, empyema, pneumothorax, Pancoast's tumor, gallbladder disease, peptic ulcer, diaphragmatic hernia, subphrenic abscess, and perisplenitis. Causalgic pain must be differentiated from somatic pain when involvement of the autonomic nervous system may be the cause of the symptoms. The recognition of a neuropathic joint, which, contrary to the usual teaching, is by no means necessarily painless, may lead to the diagnosis of a disease such as syringomyelia, neurosyphilis, or diabetes.

Finally, although joint pain may be arising primarily from joint dysfunction, the pain in the joint may persist in spite of adequate treatment because of a secondary low-grade infective arthritis arising from some distant focus of infection such as teeth, tonsils, sinuses, and the genitourinary or gastrointestinal tracts, symptoms of which may be revealed during discussion of the patient's system review.

OBSERVATIONS FROM CLINICAL EXPERIENCES

There are certain interesting and peculiar features that on clinical observation may suggest the correct diagnosis of joint pain. For instance, pain that migrates from joint to joint in a patient who shows clinical evidence of systemic illness is suggestive of rheumatic fever. The single painful joint that is apparently so painful that the patient withdraws it as the examiner prepares to examine it is suggestive of the acute gonococcal joint. What appears to be a relatively mild problem in a single joint but has more marked associated muscle atrophy than expected is often the tuberculous joint. In considering the joints of the fingers, it is often said that osteoarthritis affects the distal interphalangeal joints, that rheumatoid arthritis affects the proximal interphalangeal joints, and that gout affects the metacarpophalangeal joints. Joint pain from gout is by no means limited to the feet, nor is it by any means always associated with tophi; gout may occur in any of the joints of the limbs and even in the joints of the vertebral column. The less common forms of arthritis may be suggested to the diagnostician only by the absence of the diagnostic features of the more common causes of joint pain.

The relationship of osteoarthritis to the diagnosis and treatment of joint pain is cogent to this thesis but is dealt with in Chapter 2. It is sufficient to reiterate here that a patient can have pain-free osteoarthritis for years before symptoms draw attention to it; after painful arthritis has been treated successfully, the patient once again has pain-free osteoarthritis.

Excess Fluid in a Joint

It should be possible to decide the nature of excess fluid within a synovial joint from one's initial clinical examination, not the least part of which is the history of the swelling.

Excess fluid may be due to an excess of synovial fluid, which may follow trauma or may be a manifestation of disease. It may be due to blood, which may also be caused by trauma of a more severe nature than that which causes an outpouring of synovial fluid into the joint. The clinical picture of

blood in the joint without a history of trauma is suggestive of diseases such as hemophilia and pigmented villonodular synovitis, which is a condition that falls between inflammation and neoplasm in that it is locally invasive but it does not metastasize. These two conditions are the only causes of spontaneous bleeding into a joint. The third type of fluid that may be found in a joint is pus. Blood and pus have lysins in them, which destroy hyaline cartilage; as soon as their presence is recognized, they should be aspirated.

The clinical differences among these three types of fluid are usually quite clear. The onset of traumatic synovitis is when an injury occurs with unsustained pain and is followed by a latent period of up to 24 hours before swelling becomes noticeable; the swelling may be large when the patient is first seen. Even excess synovial fluid is normal to a joint, so that it does not set up an acute inflammatory reaction. The swollen joint, therefore, is warm but not hot, and the patient complains of discomfort and stiffness rather than of pain with loss of movement. By contrast, the onset of swelling due to blood is sudden. If the clotting mechanism is normal, the swelling is relatively small. Because blood is foreign to the joint, it sets up an acute inflammatory reaction, giving rise to heat and pain; the patient complains of impaired movement.

The natural history of pus in a joint is entirely different in that its onset occurs in a patient who has been obviously sick for up to 10 days or more; the patient suddenly develops acute pain and absolute loss of movement of the involved joint and is sicker in appearance than during the incubating period. In an infant or a child, for instance, the condition is often designated a cause of pseudoparesis and is a medical emergency. Such a condition in children and infants has led to the misdiagnosis of acute poliomyelitis.

There is another condition involving the elbow of a child known as the pulled elbow. This in fact is a manifestation of acute joint dysfunction in a perfectly healthy child, the condition of which can immediately be restored to normal by manipulative therapy. The pseudoparesis of a pyarthrosis is associated with a child who has had persistent upper respiratory tract infection or unabated diarrhea (or both). Pyarthrosis of a hip is manifested by the pseudoparesis with the involved hip held immobile at a 90° angle, which is the most relaxed position of the capsule of the joint. No attempt should be made to straighten out a leg held in this manner for fear of rupturing the capsule, which could leave an individual crippled for life.

The importance of differentiating these conditions clinically is that the fluid should not be withdrawn from a joint in which there is simple synovitis, whereas the removal of blood and pus from a joint is mandatory. The reason that the joint with simple traumatic synovitis should not be aspirated is that synovial fluid is normal to a joint, and excess fluid will be absorbed normally as soon as the pathologic condition that has given rise to its excess has resolved. Its presence in excess is the best clinical indication that all is not well within the joint; if it does not disappear spontaneously, then either the diagnosis is wrong or the treatment is wrong (or both). The unnecessary introduction of needles in the joints should be avoided because of the chances of introducing infection.

The excess synovial fluid of traumatic synovitis will, of course, never disappear so long as the joint is subjected to the repetitive minor trauma of use while the active traumatic injury is present. Thus the correct treatment of traumatic synovitis is rest from function, but not rest from movement; the movement part of the treatment must never cause pain, however. This is probably the most important teaching in the treatment of any joint problem, for if this movement concept were followed more assiduously in the treatment of joints afflicted by various pathologic conditions there would be far fewer disabling residues

from joint injury. It must be made perfectly clear, however, that movement in this context may mean simply 1° or 2° of movement and by no means denotes putting the joint through anything resembling its normal range of voluntary movement.

There remain a number of clinical clues that should help a physician arrive at a correct diagnosis of joint pain; these are not necessarily accompanied by fluctuance, although discoloration and elevation of skin temperature remain obvious. The first of these is gout, which can easily be mistaken for an abscess or an infected joint. There is also an interesting relationship among muscle atrophy, joint swelling, and pain that may be useful in differentiating two other etiologic factors in acute joint pain. When a joint is infected by gonococci, exaggerated pain is characteristic, but there is little apparent joint swelling and little obvious muscle atrophy. When the examiner approaches a patient with acute gonococcal arthritis, the patient withdraws from the examining hand. In a similar way the patient withdraws from the touch of an examiner when suffering from Sudeck's bone atrophy or a limb in which there is reflex muscular dystrophy. There is also a strange combination of signs when the cause of joint disease is tuberculosis. For some reason there is unusually marked muscle atrophy with little joint swelling and an insignificant complaint of pain. Stress fractures in osteoporotic bone close to a joint may be mistaken for a primary joint inflammatory process.

Clues Suggesting Joint Dysfunction

In review, when joint dysfunction is the primary cause of joint pain, the clues in the patient's history are that the symptom of pain was sudden in onset, occurred after some unguarded joint movement, was unassociated with marked swelling or warmth, is limited to one joint, is lessened by rest (which does not produce stiffness), and is aggravated by activity.

PHYSICAL EXAMINATION

The techniques used in physical examination that are now going to be described are not meant to replace anyone's individual method of examining patients complaining of musculoskeletal pain. They are additional examination techniques to elicit physical signs by which the examiner can more predictably arrive at a diagnosis not only of the structure in the system that may be involved in pathologic change but also of the nature of the pathologic change in the structure. The reader is referred to Table 3-2, in which history taking is stressed as being almost the most important part of the clinical investigation of the patient complaining of musculoskeletal pain. Short cuts in this requirement in the practice of medicine can only result in errors of diagnosis.

General Physical Examination

Temperature and Pulse

The patient's temperature and the pulses of all four limbs should be noted before any examination of a pain problem in the musculoskeletal system is undertaken. A patient complaining of musculoskeletal pain who is running a fever or has unequal or irregular pulses probably should not be put through the stress of further physical examination of the musculoskeletal system until the cause of these abnormalities has been determined.

Inspection

Any painful area should be inspected before it is palpated or moved. The color of

the skin and the presence or absence of localized or generalized swelling should be noted. The alteration of muscle contour or noticeable muscle atrophy is important. The affected limb or area of the back should always be compared to the side of the body that is pain free.

Palpation

Before any part of the system is moved at all, it should be palpated at rest. At this time differences of local skin temperature may be appreciated, and the presence of fluctuation within a joint, the consistency of the synovial capsule of the joint, and the consistency of the supporting and mobilizing muscles of the joint must all be noted. Let the examiner always be aware that the lighter the touch, the more can be felt. If an occult fracture of a long bone is suspected as a possible cause of pain, it is at this time that the sound conduction of the bone on the pain-free side is assessed before this examination is repeated on the painful side. If an aspiration of the injured part is contemplated to see whether there is any fat floating on the aspirated fluid, this is the time to do it.

If, for instance, a knee joint that by history is limited in movement is painful after the healing of a fracture of one of the bones of the leg, and if there is obvious fibrosis and binding down of the quadriceps expansion (which is invariably associated with atrophy of the quadriceps), it should be immediately obvious that the patella is fixed in its cephalad range of movement. In this position, the patella blocks flexion of the knee, and it is impossible to restore movement to the knee joint until the patella is mobilized. Nor, in these circumstances, can it be anticipated that normal physiology can be restored to the quadriceps muscle until the fibrotic changes in the quadriceps expansion are reversed. Mobilizing procedures to the joint or an exercise program for the muscle must fail.

The ligaments of the joint being examined must all be palpated individually because it is classic that ligaments are never tender unless they are torn or ruptured or unless there is some pathologic condition within the joint that they support. It should also be remembered that the normal capsule of a joint cannot be appreciated by palpation. If the capsule can be palpated, then there is some pathologic condition within the joint or in the capsule itself.

Because we are dealing with a system, and because we have talked of the patella being bound down, it is useful to remember that there is no muscle designed to pull the patella caudally. This lost patella movement is truly a lost movement of joint play because it can only be restored by manual manipulative means. A prerequisite for normal function is normal joint play. Besides there being no muscle to restore the functional position of the patella in relation to the femoral condyles and to the superpatellar pouch of the capsule, there is muscle to which little attention is paid. This is the genu articularis, which pulls the upper pole of the capsule up the leg so that it is not pinched between the femur and the patella in normal functional movement. It is logical to suppose that this muscle, which has no distal fixed attachment, becomes bound up in this scarring of the quadriceps mechanism, loses its muscle characteristics, and becomes fibrotic from disuse atrophy. It does not, however, become a pain-free structure, and it is constantly being pinched between the patella and the femur during function, so that chronic pain ensues.

It is not beyond the realm of common sense to look at the small, untrained, disused muscles in the back. We refer to the rotatores and the intertransversalis muscles, which, once they are involved in a damaged area of the spine, cannot be restored to their normal function and must interfere with a retraining program. One further example of the problems of restoration becomes apparent when one considers that a child born without arms can be taught to do virtually anything that a normal child can do but with its feet instead of with its hands. This is extremely difficult in an adult because disuse, immobilization in shoes, and neglect produce irreversible changes in the muscles that make them untrainable and also because the deconditioning is a factor that produces joint dysfunction and pain in any of the joints that normally might be used.

Examination of Movements in the Voluntary Range

In the presence of signs of active inflammation within the joint, which can be detected by the examination procedures described up to this point, it is unnecessary to examine joint movement at all. Examination of joint movement in infants under these conditions may indeed be disastrous.

In the absence of signs of active inflammation within the joint, movement of the joint in its voluntary range should be noted as it is performed actively by the patient and then should be checked by passive examination. The degrees of movement in each normal range of movement should be noted as a baseline from which improvement or deterioration can be checked and also for comparison with the unaffected side. When the pain is in a joint of one of the lower extremities, any inequality of leg length should be noted because this may cause unnatural stresses of weight bearing at otherwise normal joints and may result in joint dysfunction from relatively innocuous unguarded movements. It also may result in early changes of traumatic osteoarthritis, or it may cause laxity of the supporting ligaments from constant repetitive strain from otherwise normal function. Any insufficiency of the Achilles tendons should be noted; the importance of Achilles tendon insufficiency is discussed in some detail in Chapter 5.

Gait

Study of the gait may prove to be an important aid in diagnosis. A gluteus medius gait is commonly associated with pathologic changes in the hip joint, for instance. It should be remembered that the examination of a painful knee joint is incomplete until the hip joint on the same side has been examined also. Any child complaining of pain in the knee must be assumed to have a pathologic condition in the hip on the same side until it is proved otherwise. Some neurologic diseases have characteristic gaits.

Muscle Examination

The mobilizing and stabilizing muscles of the involved joint must then be examined. Muscle atrophy may be appreciated by inspection, but it can also be checked quite accurately in certain situations by measurements. In considering knee joint pain, it is particularly important to assess atrophy of the vastus medialis accurately. In the average patient, circumferential measurement of the thigh 2 inches above the patella detects masked synovial swelling in the suprapatellar pouch. Circumferential measurement of the thigh 4 inches above the patella specifically detects atrophy of the vastus medialis, which is invariably present with pathologic conditions of the knee joint. Measurement of the circumference of the thigh more proximal to this point detects group muscle atrophy, which is more commonly associated with pathologic conditions of the spine. As long as there is any atrophy or weakness of a vastus medialis muscle, the knee will remain unstable, even after the successful treatment and eradication of any pathologic cause of pain within the knee joint. Because the vastus medialis comes into full play only in the last 15° of voluntary extension of the knee joint, reeducative exercises

prescribed for the quadriceps muscles often fail to restore normal strength and function to the vastus medialis because of the inadequate way in which a patient is taught to do the exercises. Too often the importance of the last 15° of movement is not stressed, so that the patient fails to concentrate on completing full extension.

Muscle weakness may occur without atrophy, although this is unlikely. A manual muscle test is often an important part of the clinical examination and provides another baseline from which improvement or deterioration of a pathologic condition in the joint may be assessed. Electrical muscle tests are of value only when some interruption of the neuromuscular mechanism is suspected. Muscle volume and power should always be compared with those on the unaffected side.

Measurements of leg length are also rather carelessly performed, often through some sort of clothing and often with a tape crossing over the patella in an oblique manner, making it impossible to compare future measurements when they are made or if they are made by a different examiner. Further, these measurements must be made between fixed bony points. One end of the tape is fixed under the anterior-superior iliac spine, and the other end is fixed under the tip of the medial malleolus. If this length of tape is now transferred to the opposite limb without any reference being made to the markings on the tape, a difference of length can accurately be run off by the thumb which is in relation to the medial malleolus.

Reference has been made earlier to making a measurement between the posterior superior iliac spines. For this to be accurate the ends of the tape must be fixed. They are hooked medially around the bony prominences. Measuring their distance by placing the tape *over* the prominences destroys the worth of comparing this measurement in a patient sitting and prone because the tape cannot be between fixed points with any certainty. The absence of movement between the posterior superior iliac spines with change of posture is pathognomonic of disease of the sacroiliac joint.

AUXILIARY EXAMINATIONS

The habit of ordering auxiliary examinations before examining the patient must be deprecated. The various high-tech examinations show changes that are too frequently blamed for symptoms because there is no way of knowing when such changes first occur.

Obvious radiographic joint changes cannot suddenly have appeared from an injury sustained the day before the picture is taken, nor will the changes alter if the symptoms disappear through one or another therapeutic endeavor. The obvious exception to this is the presence of a fracture: Even a new fracture may not show up radiographically for a week or two after the injury. For this reason the causes of symptoms are frequently overlooked. One instance of this was a patient who had been fused a week earlier for pain arising from spondylolisthesis when in fact the pathologic source of pain was tuberculosis at the T-11 junction. For the most part, radiographs and the various scans that are now available should be used to confirm a clinical diagnosis, not to make it.

There are no characteristic changes in joints to suggest the diagnosis of joint dysfunction, and joint dysfunction may be the cause of symptoms in the absence of any abnormal radiographic changes at all. Many errors could be avoided if radiologists resumed their clinical assessment of patients who are being radiologically examined, and often the radiologist should consult with the referring physician before making any conclusive report.

Sometimes special X-ray techniques are needed before an accurate diagnosis of joint pathology can be arrived at. Stress radiographs may have to be taken to determine the integrity of the supporting ligaments of a joint. Stereoscopic films may help determine the localization of loose bodies within the joint. Depth estimations may have to be made by the radiologist to determine whether foreign bodies are intraarticular or extraarticular. Some advocate the use of arthrograms, and certainly they may be useful diagnostically, especially in determining the presence of a tear in a joint capsule, in which case a radiopaque dye is injected into the joint. In some instances the presence of traumatic injury of an intraarticular fibrocartilage can be determined when air is used as the contrast medium.

LABORATORY PROCEDURES

There are no laboratory data that are characteristic of the common or garden-variety aches and pains arising from the musculoskeletal system. The fact that the serum calcium and phosphorus levels, when multiplied together, is usually 40 mg/dL in patients who do not suffer from problems in the musculoskeletal system, and that this figure is close to 30 mg/dL in patients who do have musculoskeletal problems, is just an empirical observation, and doubtless this might represent a fertile field for research. The fact that the sweat of a patient is acidic when he or she is suffering from many musculoskeletal problems and returns to neutral on healing is empirical also, but this, too, might represent a fertile field for research. The fact that most patients who suffer from simple musculoskeletal problems have a deficient fluid intake is also an empirical observation but could be another basis for research.

Nevertheless, certain laboratory tests can be quite specific as accurate aids in the differential diagnosis of the causes of joint pain. A complete blood count and erythrocyte sedimentation rate should be routine. Many patients with musculoskeletal symptoms show a deficiency type of anemia, and many show a relative lymphocytosis. A determination of the serum uric acid may lead to a diagnosis of gout. An estimation of the albumin-globulin ratio and the performance of the usual complement fixation tests, flocculation tests, and agglutination tests may be necessary before conditions such as rheumatoid arthritis, brucellosis, typhoid fever, or syphilis, for instance, may be diagnosed or ruled out.

Hematologic study for lupus erythematosus may be necessary, and such nonspecific determinations as the C-reactive protein may be useful in conjunction with other laboratory data. Certainly, serial determinations of the antistreptolysin O titer may be essential in revealing rheumatic fever and in following the activity of the disease. The heterophile antibody may reveal infectious mononucleosis to be the underlying problem. Sickle cell disease in an Afro-American patient may give the clue to the correct diagnosis. Parasitic ova may have to be sought in the stools. Urinalysis, urine culture, and such things as throat culture and blood cultures may have to be done. Skin tests may also be necessary.

A painful joint may have to be aspirated for diagnostic purposes. The cellular content of synovial fluid may give a clue to the pathologic condition within the joint, and the synovial fluid may have to be cultured to determine the organism causing infection and its sensitivity to antibiotics. There are times when synovial biopsy is essential to arrive at a correct diagnosis of the cause of joint pain. Lyme disease and AIDS have to be added to the long list of causes of acute pain in the musculoskeletal system.

EXAMINATION FOR MOVEMENTS OF JOINT PLAY

Although it is true that many of the foregoing auxiliary diagnostic procedures are often unnecessary and even redundant in arriving at the correct diagnosis of the cause

of pain in the musculoskeletal system, they have been discussed in this order to reemphasize the fact that joint dysfunction and muscle trigger points are but additional diagnostic conclusions to be arrived at in assessing a problem of joint pain. By the same token, it should not be forgotten that it is also pertinent to this thesis that joint dysfunction is one of the commonest causes of joint pain in clinical medicine. Evidence of joint dysfunction is therefore sought early in the absence of any clinical signs to suggest more serious joint disease.

Rules for Joint Play Examination

To examine for joint play movements, the patient must be recumbent; only in this position does the examiner have perfect control of the examining movements that are being performed. The only exception to this is in the examination of the joints of the fingers and the wrists. The position of examination is vital to the accumulation of precise data relating to joint movement. The techniques of eliciting normal joint play must be adhered to. It must be remembered that the movements of joint play are in a passive range. Each is usually less than ⅛ inch in extent. Their performance requires accuracy and precision. Rules for joint play examination are detailed in Chapter 3.

Exceptions to Rules of Joint Play Examination

In the following chapters, which describe topographically the specific manipulation techniques used in the assessment of painful joints when searching for evidence of joint dysfunction, it will be noted that rule 3 (examining one joint at a time) and rule 4 (examining one movement at each joint at a time) are frequently broken. For example, the examining maneuver for eliciting long axis extension of the midcarpal joint, the radiocarpal joint, and the ulnomeniscotriquetral joint, as well as the maneuver for pulling the head of the radius downward on the ulna at the elbow, are all the same. When examining the glenohumeral joint it will be noted that the movement of long axis extension at the midcarpal and radiocarpal joints is being performed. Coincidentally, while the head of the humerus is pulled downward in the glenoid cavity the play movements of long axis extension of the joints distal to the shoulder are all going into long axis extension.

Incidentally, it may seem that the identical manipulative maneuver is being used for examination of long axis extension at the mortise joint and the subtalar joint. However, it is not the case. In the former, the web between the examiner's thumb and index finger of the right hand is over the neck of the talus. In the latter it is over the navicula. The left-hand web does remain over the Achilles tubercle when performing the talar rock and the medial and lateral tilt movements of the calcaneus on the talus.

With regard to the examination of the joints of the upper limbs, it is surprising how seldom both the midcarpal and the radiocarpal joints are affected at the same time by joint dysfunction from any cause. In searching for impairment of the long axis extension at either joint, one is simply taking up the slack of normal long axis extension of the uninvolved joint to determine its presence or absence in the other joint. If dysfunction is present in both joints, then the mechanical diagnosis of pain is unlikely. Rarely is there clinical evidence of loss of the joint play movement of long axis extension at the ulnomeniscotriquetral joint. This presumably is because the articulating surfaces of the two bones are separated relatively widely by the intraarticular meniscus.

The downward movement of the head of the radius on the ulna, which is accomplished by using the same technique, is legitimate if there is no pathologic involvement of the midcarpal or radiocarpal joints. The performance of these movements is simply part of taking up the slack before exerting the manipulative pull to move the head of the radius. The same criteria hold for exerting the therapeutic manipulative maneuver of pulling the head of the humerus downward in the glenoid cavity at the maximum angle of arm abduction.

When we come to discuss long axis extension at the mortise joint and the subtalar joint in the lower extremity, the same rationalization must be allowed. It is clinically strange how often long axis extension is impaired at the subtalar joint without there being any impairment of the same movement at the mortise joint, yet if both joints are involved the mechanical diagnosis of pain is unlikely. In eliciting the joint play movements of the talar rock and side tilt medially and laterally at the subtalar joint, however, rules 3 and 4 are deliberately broken. These are the only times when this is so.

The key word in the foregoing paragraph is *deliberately*. The only time that the user of manipulative techniques may break these rules is when he or she knowingly does it for a specific reason. If the rules are broken unknowingly, damage may be inflicted upon the joint being examined. If the rules are broken unknowingly when a therapeutic manipulation is being performed, severe injury may be inflicted upon the joint being treated, and the novice will blame the procedure rather than his or her lack of knowledge of the technique for the worsening of the joint condition and the failure of the treatment to bring the patient relief.

chapter 5

Examples of Examining Procedures

I. Normal Joint Play in the Synovial Joints of the Foot

THE METATARSOPHALANGEAL AND INTERPHALANGEAL JOINTS

The range of joint play in the metatarsophalangeal joints and the interphalangeal joints is the same. The extent of each movement is different, and the facility with which the movements may be performed is limited by the anatomic structure of the soft parts of the foot. Pain from dysfunction is usually limited to the metatarsophalangeal joints. The phalangeal joints of the toes seldom are involved in pain-producing dysfunction.

For illustration purposes, the first metatarsophalangeal joint is used to illustrate normal joint play. The movements of metatarsal joint play are long axis extension, anteroposterior tilt, side tilt medially and laterally, and rotation. To illustrate this, the big toe is used. As with the metacarpophalangeal joints, a golf club grip is used to produce long axis extension of the base of the first phalanx away from the stabilized head of the first metatarsal bone. The pull is made in the direction of the phalanx as it is found with the patient at rest.

A minor change has to be made in performing this movement at the lateral four metatarsophalangeal joints because of the basic anatomy of the foot. It is not possible to use a golf club grip. Instead, a platform is made of the fully flexed index finger of the examiner's mobilizing hand, which rests under the foot as close to the base of the phalanx as possible. The thumb rests flat over the dorsum of the foot, which prevents painful pinching. The slack is taken up, and the pull is exerted in the long axis of each toe.

Long Axis Extension

The examiner holds the head of the metatarsal bone between the right thumb and index finger and grasps the base of the proximal phalanx between the left thumb and index finger. The thumb is placed on the dorsal aspect of the proximal phalanx base, and the left index finger is placed on its plantar aspect. The proximal phalanx is pulled away from the head of the metatarsal bone in the direction of the long axis of the toe. The position adopted to perform this movement is shown in Figure 5-1.

51

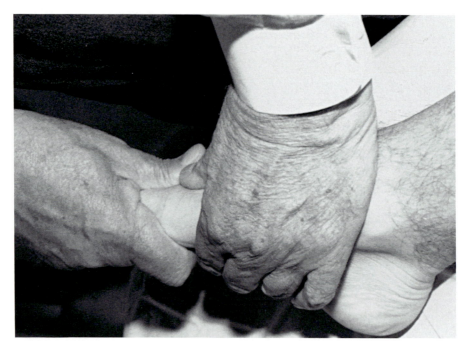

Fig. 5-1 Position adopted to perform the joint play movement of long axis extension at the first metatarsophalangeal joint.

Anteroposterior Tilt

The examiner maintains the stabilizing grip and places the tip of the left thumb just distal to the base of the proximal phalanx dorsally. The tip of the left index finger is just distal to the base of the phalanx on its plantar surface. Using the left thumb and the left index finger alternately as a fulcrum, the examiner tilts the base of the subject's phalanx alternately backward and forward. This opens the joint's dorsal and plantar aspect. Figure 5-2 illustrates the dorsal phase of this joint play movement, as well as the position adopted to elicit it. Figure 5-3 illustrates the plantar phase.

Side Tilt Medially and Laterally

The examiner maintains the stabilizing grip on the head of the metatarsal bone

with the right hand and places the tip of the left thumb deep in the web between the first and second toes and the tip of the left index finger medially just distal to the base of the proximal phalanx. The thumb is used as a pivot, and the metatarsophalangeal joint is tilted open on its medial aspect by exerting pressure through the tip of the left index finger. Then the tip of the index finger is used as a pivot, and the metatarsophalangeal joint is tilted open laterally by exerting pressure through the thumb. Figure 5-4 illustrates the position at the completed phase of the lateral side tilt joint play movement. Figure 5-5 illustrates the side tilt medially. There is a mobilizing force in both finger and thumb in each movement.

Rotation

The examiner maintains the grip on the head of the metatarsal bone with the left

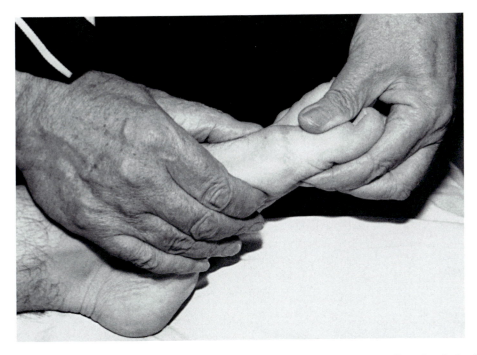

Fig. 5-2 Dorsal phase of tilting open the first metatarsophalangeal joint. The tilt is achieved by using the lumbrical muscle of the index finger, the tip of which is placed as close to the base of the phalanx as possible.

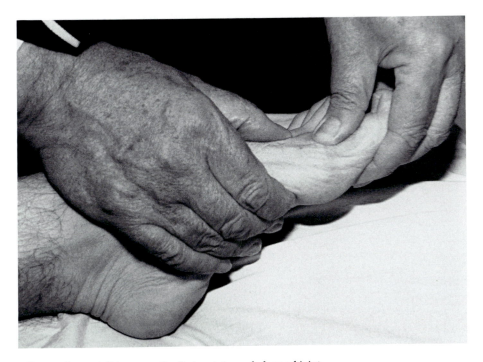

Fig. 5-3 Plantar phase of tilting open the first metatarsophalangeal joint.

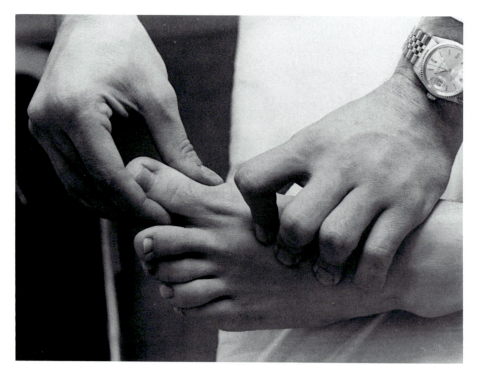

Fig. 5-4 Position at the completed phase of the lateral side tilt joint play movement.

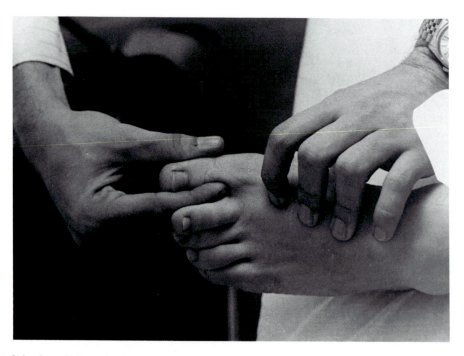

Fig. 5-5 Side tilt medially at the first metatarsal joint.

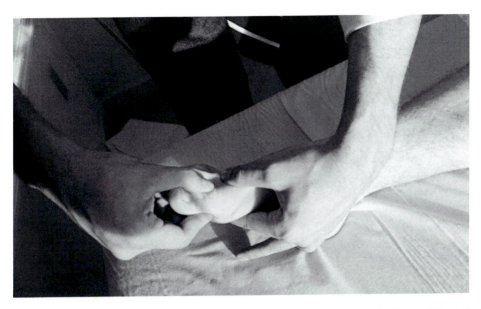

Fig. 5-6 Rotation of the base of the phalanx on the head of the metatarsal bone of the big toe. The shaft of the phalanx is protected from torque if the thumb and second and third fingers of the examiner's right hand are close enough to the base of the bone.

hand and grasps the proximal phalanx with the right thumb, index finger, and middle finger, hooking the distal phalanx of the fourth and fifth fingers on the lateral aspect of the subject's distal flexed phalanx. The examiner rotates the proximal phalanx on the metatarsal head clockwise and counterclockwise in its long axis. Figure 5-6 shows the position adopted to elicit this movement.

The joint play movements of the other metatarsophalangeal and interphalangeal joints are elicited in the same way, only the degree of normal movement being different.

THE DISTAL INTERMETATARSAL JOINTS

The movements of joint play between the heads of each metatarsal bone are anteroposterior glide and rotation. The joints between these bones are not true synovial joints anatomically, but functionally the movement between them may be impaired. If dysfunction occurs, the symptoms of pain are produced just as though they were synovial joints. The stationary axis is the second metatarsophalangeal complex.

Anteroposterior Glide

With the subject in the recumbent position, the examiner sits at the end of the table facing the plantar aspect of the subject's foot (the left foot is used for illustration). The examiner grasps the neck of the second metatarsal bone, the right thumb being on the plantar aspect and the fingers on the dorsal aspect. The examiner grasps the metatarsal bone of the first toe in a similar manner with the left hand. The second metatarsal bone is stabilized, and the head of the first metatarsal bone is moved upward and downward upon it. The reader should remember that the words *upward* and *downward* are used in an anatomic sense; the movement of the heads of the metatarsal bones is positionally forward and backward.

The role of the examiner's hands is then reversed. The examiner grasps the second metatarsal bone with the left hand, and with the right (mobilizing) hand moves the head of the third metatarsal bone upward and downward upon it as illustrated. The examiner then stabilizes the third metatarsal bone with the left hand, and with the right hand moves the head of the fourth metatarsal bone upward and downward upon it. Finally, the fourth metatarsal bone is stabilized with the examiner's left hand, and the head of the fifth metatarsal bone is moved upward and downward upon it. Figure 5-7 shows the movement of the head of the fifth metatarsal bone upon the fourth.

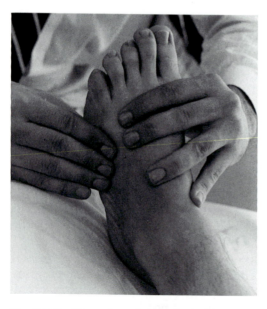

Fig. 5-7 Position adopted to perform the anteroposterior glide between the heads of the fourth and fifth metatarsal bones. The fourth metatarsal is stabilized.

Rotation

The examiner grasps the neck of the first metatarsal bone between the left thumb and index finger, which are placed at right angles to the shaft of the metatarsal bone. With a wrist flexion, the examiner rotates the head of the first metatarsal bone in the long axis of its shaft clockwise and counterclockwise upon the head of the second metatarsal bone.

The role of the examiner's hands is then reversed, the left hand now stabilizing the second metatarsal bone. The neck of the third metatarsal bone is grasped between the examiner's right thumb and index finger, which are placed at right angles to its long axis, and with a wrist flexion it is rotated clockwise and counterclockwise on the stabilized head of the second metatarsal bone. The examiner then stabilizes the third metatarsal bone with the left hand, and with the right hand rotates the head of the fourth metatarsal bone on the head of the third. The examiner finally stabilizes the fourth metatarsal bone and rotates the head of the fifth metatarsal bone on the head of the fourth. Figure 5-8 illustrates the rotary movement of the head of the fifth metatarsal bone on that of the fourth.

THE TARSOMETATARSAL JOINTS

The joint play movements of the tarsometatarsal joints are anteroposterior glide and rotation.

Anteroposterior Glide

The distal tarsal bones are the first, second, and third cuneiforms and the cuboid;

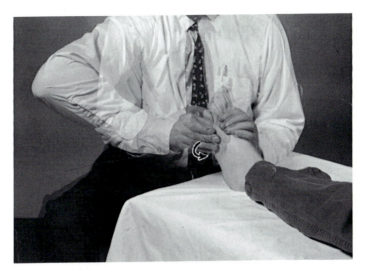

Fig. 5-8 Rotary movement of joint play of the head of the fifth metatarsal on that of the fourth metatarsal.

these are stabilized (the left foot is used for illustration). The bases of the metatarsal bones are grasped over their dorsal aspect by the examiner's right hand while the left hand stabilizes the distal tarsal bones. The mobilizing right hand alternately thrusts upward and downward, performing an anteroposterior glide movement (supero-inferior in direction) between the base of the metatarsal bones and the adjacent tarsal bones. Figures 5-9 and 5-10 illustrate this movement. The base of the fifth metatarsal bone can be moved independently on the cuboid bone to elicit the anteroposterior glide in this joint.

Rotation

There is a different degree of rotation of the bases of the metatarsal bones on their adjacent tarsal bones, and the movement cannot specifically be elicited at each joint. It has to be performed at all the joints at once. The examiner stabilizes the tarsal

bones in the manner described above (the right foot is used for illustration) and cradles the necks of the metatarsal bones with the right thumb, which is placed across them on their plantar surface (Fig. 5-11).

MIDTARSAL JOINTS

The stabilizing hand over the distal row of carpal bones remains in place. The other mobilizing hand is placed so that the examiner's index finger knuckles are touching on the medial aspect of the foot and the tips of the thumbs are touching on the outer side of the foot. Figure 5-9 reveals an open V over the dorsum of the foot; this bears no relation to the plane of the joints, which are to be moved in an anteroposterior manner. This V has to be closed by bringing the mobilizing hand proximally to the stabilizing hand. This position is illustrated in Figure 5-10. The anteroposterior glide is performed upward and downward, with the mobilizing hand rubbing against the

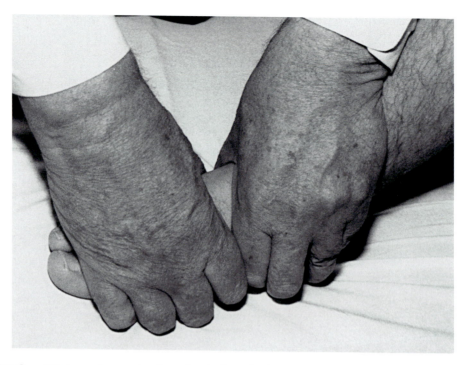

Fig. 5-9 Open V between the examiner's two hands above the dorsum. This is the V that has to be closed so that when the mobilizing hand moves against the stabilizing hand the force is in the right plane between these two rows of bones.

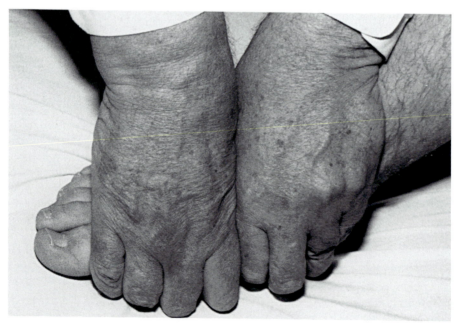

Fig. 5-10 Examiner's hands together after closing the V. The anteroposterior glide is achieved through shoulder movements transmitted through the straight arm onto the bases of the metatarsal bones, first upward and then rebounding downward.

A

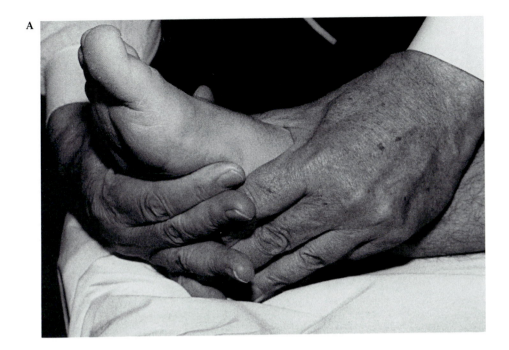

B

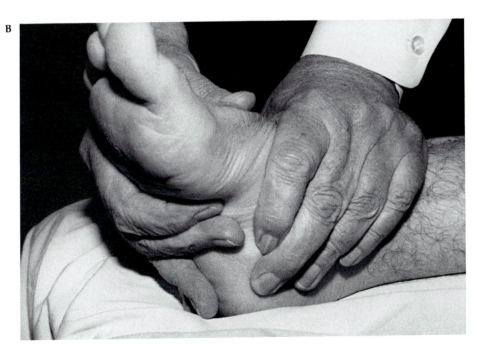

Fig. 5-11 (A) Position adopted to perform the rotary movements between the bases of the metatarsal bones on the distal row of tarsal bones. (B) The left hand stabilizes the three cuneiforms and the cuboid. The right hand is the mobilizing hand. Both take up the slack in the way in which one wrings out a towel. When all the slack is taken up, the right hand moves in the same arc of the circle, performing the normal play movement. (C) The hands are positioned in the same way as for B. The slack is taken up in a wringing movement in the opposite direction to that in B. When all the slack is taken up, the right hand continues in the same arc of the circle, performing the normal play movement in the counterclockwise direction.

C

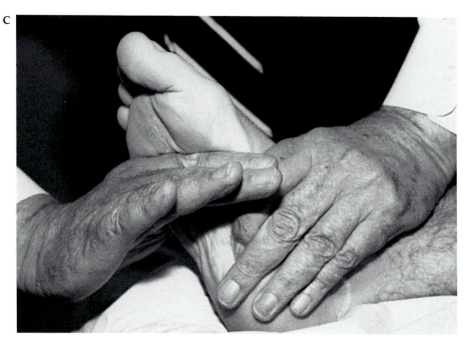

Fig 5-11 *continued*

---

stabilizing hand. The excursion of the movement is less than ½ inch now in the correct plane of the joint.

Navicula-Cuneiform Joint

There is one play movement in this joint. It is an anteroposterior (superioinferior) movement of the three cuneiform bones on the navicula (scaphoid). The examiner stabilizes the navicula and cuboid with the left hand over the dorsal aspect and grasps the three cuneiform bones with the right hand, moving them upward and downward alternately. Figure 5-12 illustrates the positions of the hands. The examiner alternates dorsal and plantar movement glides of the navicula and cuboid on the stabilized talus and calcaneus.

The Cuboid and Navicula on the Calcaneus and Talus

The anterior phase of the anteroposterior movements of the navicula on the talus and the cuboid on the calcaneus is well elicited by the examining maneuver used to demonstrate long axis extension at the subtalar (subastragaloid) joint. Figure 5-13 shows radiographically the extent to which the navicula and the cuboid move.

INTERTARSAL JOINTS

There is joint play movement (superioinferior in direction) between each tarsal bone. This cannot be appreciated clinically

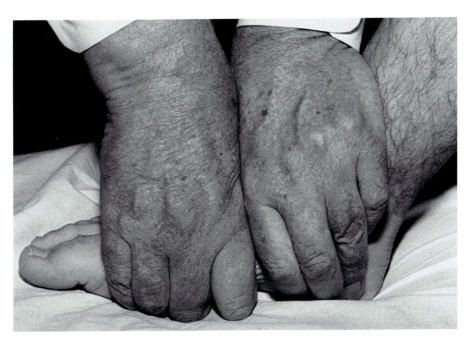

Fig. 5-12 Position adopted to perform the anteroposterior glide of the cuneiform bones on the navicula. Refer to Figure 5-10, in which less of the big toe is visible.

on examination unless there has been a traumatic subluxation of one of the bones upon another. The subluxation is usually upward, and there is a clinical sign of pain on pressing the affected bone downward on examination. The range of the specific play movement consists of each bone's moving slightly upward upon its neighbor.

THE JOINTS OF THE ANKLE

There are two major joints at the ankle. These are the mortise and the subtalar joints. To differentiate mortise joint pain from subtalar joint pain, three clinical tests are available.

The clue to the mortise joint being the source of pain is passive movement, as illustrated in Figure 5-14. The examiner's left hand elicits the movements of dorsiflexion and plantar flexion. If these movements are free from pain, the mortise joint is not the pain source.

If the examiner ceases to guide the forefoot with the right hand but continues to push the foot forward from the tibia, the added extent of movement is because the talus rocks forward on the calcaneus (Fig. 5-15). Pain in this new range suggests the subtalar joint as the source. This movement is not one of hyperflexion, which would only put an abnormal stretch upon the anterior transverse ligament of the ankle joint.

The talus having no muscle attachments to perform functional movement, all movements of the talus on the calcaneus are play movements. It is this rocking movement that takes up all the stresses and strains of

A

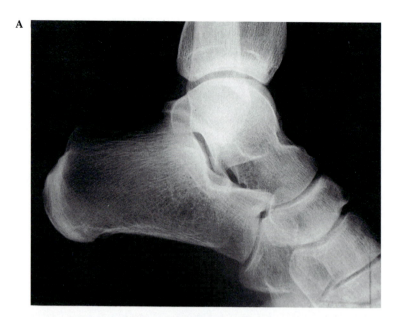

B

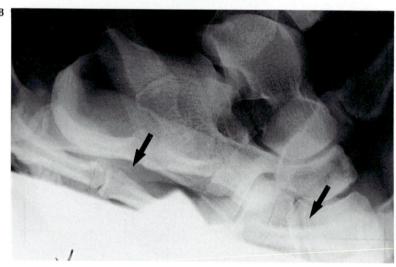

Fig. 5-13 **(A)** Lateral radiograph of a normal ankle joint at rest. The appearance of the subtalar (subastragaloid) joint should be kept in mind when studying the illustrations of joint play movement at this important joint. **(B)** Subtalar (subastragaloid) joint at the completion of the joint play movement of long axis extension. The arrows indicate the direction of the thrusts of the examiner's hands.

stubbing the toes. It spares the ankle from gross trauma both at toeoff and at heel strike. If it were not for this involuntary rocking motion at the subtalar joint, fracture dislocations around the ankle would be commonplace.

The third clinical differentiation is by ligament palpation. At the base of the sinus tarsi there is a ligament whose only function is to support the subtalar joint. If it is tender on palpation, the subtalar joint is the source of pain.

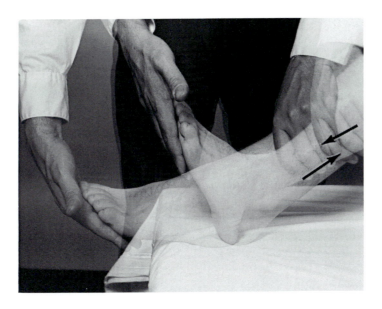

Fig. 5-14 Examining position adopted to elicit pure dorsiflexion and plantar flexion at the mortise joint. The double exposure illustrates the extent of this voluntary movement. The examiner's left hand elicits the movement by rocking the foot on the posteroinferior angle of the calcaneus. The right hand simply maintains the sole of the foot in its unchanging plane.

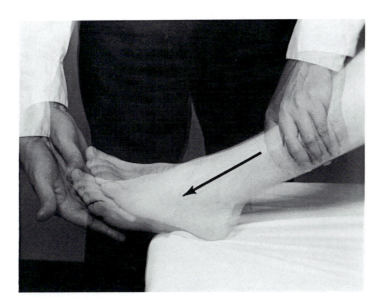

Fig. 5-15 Additional movement of apparent plantar flexion that is obtained when the joint play talar rock is brought into play. The examiner thrusts down the long axis of the tibia with the left hand (arrow) through the limit of plantar flexion, which is illustrated in Figure 5-14. The double exposure shows how the foot slips forward slightly on the couch, indicating that this is not forced plantar flexion. The examiner's right hand simply guides the foot in an unchanging plane.

The Mortise Joint

The mortise joint is made up of the lower tibial condyle and the medial malleoli. There are two movements of joint play at this joint: long axis extension and anteroposterior glide.

Long Axis Extension

The examiner sits on the couch with the back to the subject, who is lying supine. The subject's hip is abducted and flexed to not less than 90°. The knee is also flexed to a right angle. The examiner grasps the lower leg around the ankle, the left thenar web being placed posteriorly to the Achilles tendon and the right thenar web being placed over the neck of the talus, which must be clearly identified. The examiner then leans backward on the subject's thigh while pushing the foot away in the long axis of the lower leg, maintaining the foot at a right angle to it. Figure 5-16 illustrates the position adopted for the examining maneuver, and the double exposure shows the extent of the movement of long axis extension.

Anteroposterior Glide

With the subject recumbent and the hip, knee, and ankle all at 90° angles, the examiner, standing in front of the patient, grasps the subject's lower leg around the ankle above the malleoli with the left hand and the dorsum of the foot with the right hand, which stabilizes it during the performance of this movement. The mobilizing left hand then pulls forward and guides backward alternately, moving the mortise forward and backward upon the stabilized superior talar facet. Figure 5-17 shows the position adopted for eliciting this movement.

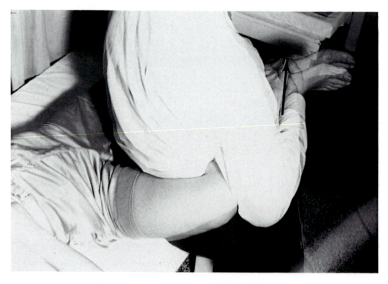

Fig. 5-16 Position adopted to elicit the joint play movement of long axis extension at the mortise joint. Note that the hip, knee, and ankle are held at right angles. The examiner thrusts forward in the long axis of the tibia, exerting countertraction by leaning backward against the posterior aspect of the subject's thigh. Note that the thrust of the examiner's hands is through the web between the thumb and index finger, over the neck of the talus. The double exposure illustrates the extent of the joint play movement of long axis extension.

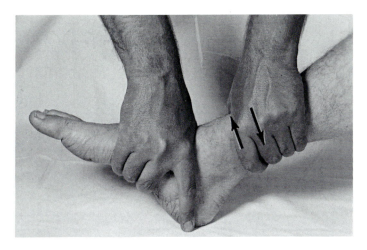

Fig. 5-17 Position adopted to elicit the anteroposterior glide of the articulating surfaces of the tibia and fibula on the talus. The examiner's left hand is the mobilizing hand. Note that the foot is held at right angles to the lower leg by the examiner's right (stabilizing) hand; the subject's knee and hip are flexed.

The Subtalar (Subastragaloid) Joint

The joint play movements at the subtalar joint are long axis extension, rock of talus on calcaneus, side tilt medially, and side tilt laterally.

Long Axis Extension

The examiner adopts the previous examining position for eliciting the joint play movement of long axis extension at the mortise joint, except for one important feature. The web of the right thumb, instead of being over the neck of the talus, is placed forward over the navicula. This allows long axis extension to leave the talus behind. Figure 5-18 illustrates the position adopted for eliciting long axis extension.

Rock of Talus on Calcaneus

The previous description of the talar rock was limited to its examination while the foot and ankle are in function. The position adopted by the examiner is the same as that used for eliciting the movement of long axis extension. In reproducing the joint play movement of the talar rock, it is necessary to perform two joint play movements at the same time. The talar rock cannot be performed passively unless the joint is in the position of long axis extension.

Holding the foot and leg with the subtalar joint in the position of the limit of long axis extension, the examiner pushes upward and forward with the hand that is behind the Achilles tendon. This rocks the calcaneus forward on the talus (Fig. 5-19). The examiner then produces the posterior rock of the talus on the calcaneus by pushing backward and downward with the hand over the dorsum of the foot (Fig. 5-20). Figures 5-21 and 5-22 are radiographs taken at the completion of the forward and backward phases of the talar rock.

These movements have nothing to do with the movements of plantar flexion and dorsiflexion, as must be studiously noted. This rocking movement of the subtalar joint

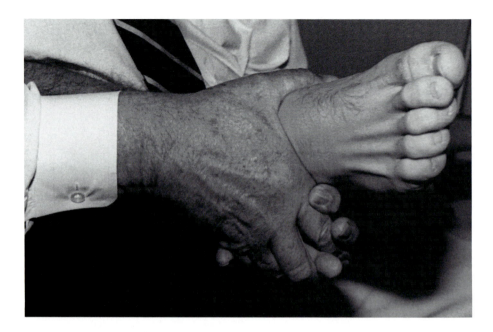

Fig. 5-18 Position adopted to elicit the joint play movement of long axis extension at the subtalar joint. It is exactly the same as that in Figure 5-16, which illustrates long axis extension at the mortise joint, except that the examiner's right hand has moved forward on the foot, so that the web between the thumb and index finger is now over the navicula. The extent of the range of this movement is, of course, a summation of long axis extension at both the mortise and the subtalar joints.

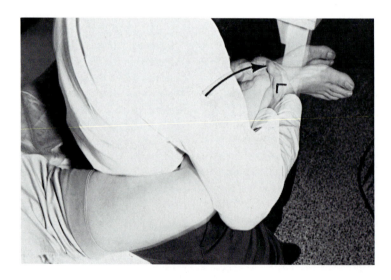

Fig. 5-19 Extent of the forward movement of the calcaneus on the talus, which is the posterior phase of the talar rock. Note that movement is elicited while full long axis extension at the mortise and subtalar joints is maintained. The examiner's left hand acts as the mobilizer (arrow), pressure being exerted on the posterior aspect of the calcaneus by the web between the thumb and index finger.

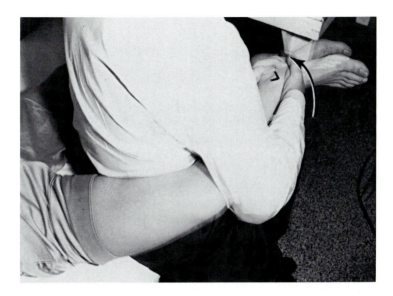

Fig. 5-20 Extent of the backward movement of the calcaneus on the talus, which is the anterior phase of the talar rock. Note that movement is elicited while full long axis extension at the mortise and subtalar joints is maintained. The examiner's right (mobilizing) hand is exerting pressure indirectly on the anterior aspect of the calcaneus through the other tarsal bones by the web between the thumb and index finger.

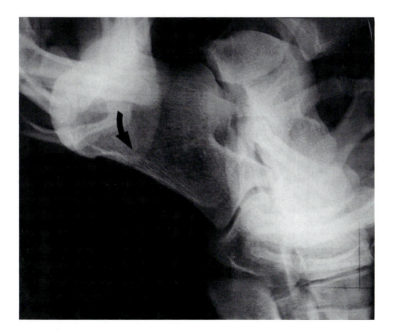

Fig. 5-21 Subtalar joint at the completion of the posterior phase of the talar rock. The arrow indicates the direction of the thrust of the examiner's hand over the posterior aspect of the calcaneus. This radiograph corresponds to the foot in Figure 5-19.

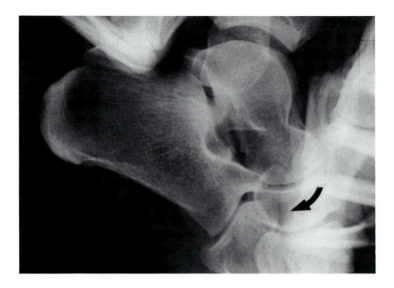

Fig. 5-22 Subtalar joint at the completion of the anterior phase of the talar rock. The arrow indicates the direction of the thrust of the examiner's hand indirectly through the other tarsal bones over the anterior aspect of the calcaneus. This movement corresponds with that illustrated in Figure 5-20.

is best appreciated by comparing the feeling of it with that of the dorsiflexion and plantar flexion movements that take place at the mortise joint.

Side Tilt Medially

The position adopted to elicit the tilting movements of the subtalar joint is the same as that adopted to produce the subtalar rock. The tilting movements can only be achieved when the joint is at the limit of long axis extension. To elicit the movement of side tilt medially, first long axis extension is performed as illustrated in Figure 5-16. When long axis extension is achieved, the examiner's thumbs are placed on the medial aspect of the calcaneus and thrust laterally, tilting the subtalar joint open on its medial aspect. This movement is a pure tilt of the calcaneus upon the talus and is not eversion of the foot at the subtalar joint.

The extent of this movement is shown in Figure 5-23.

Side Tilt Laterally

This movement is elicited in exactly the same way as the movement of medial side tilt. Instead of the tilting thrust being produced through the thumbs on the medial aspect of the calcaneus, the tilting thrust is imparted through the fingers, which are placed over the lateral aspect of the calcaneus. Figure 5-24 shows the extent of this movement.

In performing the medial tilt, the examiner uses an ulnar deviation flick equally with both hands, throwing the foot toward the ground while supporting the leg. The foot must not twist. Lateral tilt is performed by using a radial deviation flick. The examiner supports the foot and throws the leg toward the ground.

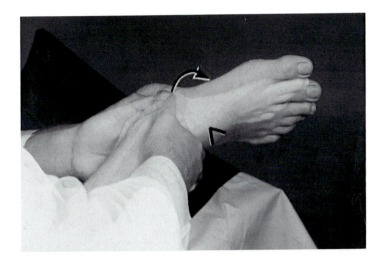

Fig. 5-23 Movement of medial side tilt of the calcaneus upon the talus, which tilts open the subtalar joint on its medial aspect. Note that movement is elicited while full long axis extension at the mortise and subtalar joints is maintained. The thrusting force (arrow) is through the examiner's thumbs on the medial aspect of the calcaneus. The fingers laterally are used as a pivot. The double exposure illustrates the extent of the movement.

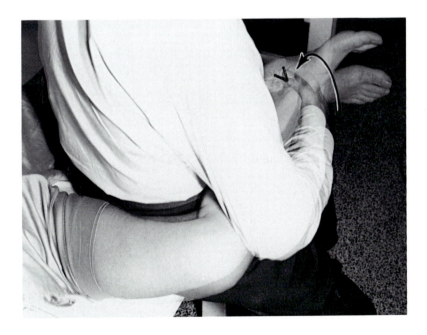

Fig. 5-24 Movement of lateral side tilt of the calcaneus upon the talus, which opens up the joint on its lateral aspect. Note that movement is elicited while full long axis extension at the mortise and subtalar joints is maintained. The thrusting force is through the fingers of both hands of the examiner on the lateral aspect of the calcaneus; medially the thumbs are used as pivots. The double exposure illustrates the extent of the movement.

THE SUPERIOR TIBIOFIBULAR JOINT

The only movement of joint play at this joint is the anteroposterior glide. If the joint play of the superior tibiofibular joint is lost and there is pain from its dysfunction, the patient may complain of pain in the knee (most often the patient complains of pain in the ankle). This is understandable when one realizes that this joint does not really play any part in the function of the knee joint proper. Minor impairment of its movement will produce greatly magnified impairment of movement of the talofibular part of the mortise joint mechanically because of the long lever arm.

The range of the joint play movement varies with the degree of knee flexion and is absent with the knee in full extension. It is maximal with the knee in midflexion.

The examiner adopts a sitting position on the subject's foot with the knee in an optimal angle of flexion. The head of the fibula is grasped between the thumb anteriorly and the tips of the index and middle fingers posteriorly. The fingers and thumb then push forward and backward alternately. The movement is not truly back and forth. The fibula head is pulled forward and guided backward (Fig. 5-25).

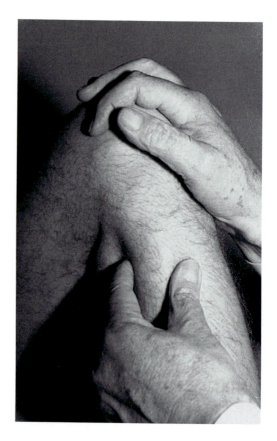

Fig. 5-25 The position adopted to elicit the antero-posterior movement at the right superior tibiofibular joint. The exposure is made at the limit of the anterior phase of the movement. The examiner's right hand stabilizes the tibia, and the left hand mobilizes the head of the fibula.

II. Normal Joint Play in the Synovial Joints of the Low Back

To emphasize that we are dealing with a system, it is not too much of a step to go from the foot and ankle to the topographic area in the back. This is a deliberate choice. The back extends from the occiput to the sacrum and includes both sacroiliac joints, the sacrococcygeal elements, and the costovertebral joints. In the low back, there are 12 interlaminar synovial joints and two sacroiliac synovial joints that must be examined for joint play. These include the joints at the thoracolumbar junction but not the coccygeal joints. There are six intervertebral discs in this area.

The range of joint play at the interlaminar joints consists of long axis extension, side tilting, and backward and forward tilting. The range of joint play movement in the sacroiliac joint is a forward and backward torsion of the ilium on the sacrum dissociated from any movement in the opposite sacroiliac joint. The patient is examined standing, sitting, supine, in the left and right side-lying positions, and prone.

STANDING

The patient stands with his or her back to the examiner and the feet together. The patient is asked to put one finger over the place that he or she considers to be the seat of pain. This localization directs attention to the probable anatomic location of pathology.

The spine is examined for any general deviation of the curves from normal and any local segmental alteration. The usual segmental change that occurs is either a flattening or a reversal of the curves or segmental scoliosis to the right or left.

The relative height of the iliac crests is noted by laying the index fingers over them, keeping the fingers parallel with the floor as illustrated in Figure 5-26.

If the crest is raised on the same side as the convexity of the scoliosis and the patient has indicated that pain is in relation to the posterior-superior iliac spine, one expects the source of pain to be the sacroiliac joint on that side.

If the iliac crest is lower on the side opposite the seat of pain and the concavity of the scoliosis is on the side of the pain, the common suspected pathology is disc prolapse or a more serious condition than joint dysfunction.

The spine is palpated with the three middle fingers of the right hand. The middle finger is placed over the spinous process and the index and ring fingers, respectively, in the right and left paraspinal troughs supporting it. The middle finger may detect a minimal vertebral rotation that it might miss if it is used alone because of the ease with which it rolls off the spinous processes.

An interspinous step discovered during this examination is characteristic of spondylolisthesis. An interspinous dip may be associated with a ruptured interspinous ligament.

Temperature changes of the skin should be noted. A sweat level change may be detected. Skin pigmentation or discoloration is diagnostically valuable. Localized swelling should be palpated and its nature assessed.

The patient is now asked to bend forward from the hips, keeping the feet together and the knees straight. (The ability or inability to touch the toes is not clinically important.) The patient should be asked to assess his or her normal degree of forward bending. This allows the physician to determine the degree of abnormality. In forward bending the whole spine should unfold in a smooth, synchronous manner. At the completion of the movement each spinous process should stand out quite distinctly, as illustrated in Figure 5-27.

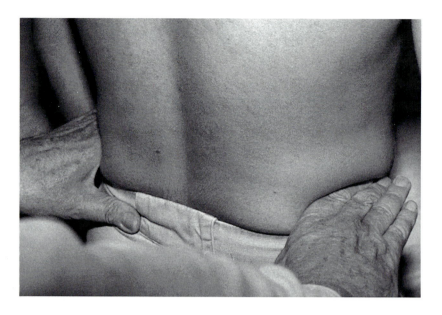

Fig. 5-26 Method used to assess the relative heights of the iliac crests with the patient standing.

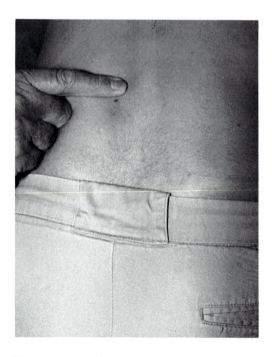

Fig. 5-27 Forward bending position. The spinous processes can be clearly seen and identified.

At the limit of forward bending, percussion over each individual vertebra should be carried out by hitting each vertebra firmly and sharply with the ulnar aspect of the closed fist. Percussion should be performed over each of the sacroiliac joints.

The patient is then asked to resume the upright position. The spine should fold up in the same smooth, synchronous manner as in unfolding.

In a condition known as flat back strain, there are two characteristic points that will suggest the diagnosis. First, the patient stoops forward with ease but complains of difficulty in regaining the upright position. Second, the symptoms of which he or she complains had their onset after deep anesthesia, usually administered for some abdominal surgery. Examination, besides revealing this difficulty of regaining the upright position, reveals a flattened lumbar lordosis that the patient cannot arch into its normal curve. There are signs of dysfunction, often at more than one level in the lumbar spine. There is abnormal movement at the intervertebral level above the flattened area.

The apparent loss of movement in the lumbar spine, which is sometimes marked, must not be confused with the loss of movement, which occurs early in cases of ankylosing spondylitis.

These are the only patient-activated voluntary movements used in this clinical examination. The other examination movements are produced passively by the examiner. The individual joint movements cannot be elicited in the presence of voluntary muscle action.

SITTING

The patient now sits on the examining table with his or her back to the examiner, the lower legs loosely hanging over the edge of the table. The patient should sit equally on both buttocks (the sparing of one buttock may be a valuable clinical sign). The curves of the spine are checked once again. Many people slouch, and their lumbar spines tend to "concertina" when sitting. This is unimportant, provided that they can resume their normal lordosis painlessly on being asked to sit up.

Measurements

Measurements should be taken before any movement. In the sitting position, the distance between the posterior-superior iliac spines is measured. This measurement should be compared with the distance between these bony points when the patient eventually assumes the prone position.

Normally there is an increase in the distance between the posterior-superior iliac spines of from ¼ to ¾ inch when measured with the patient sitting and then lying prone. In the absence of this change of distance with change of posture, there is sacroiliac joint disease. This is perhaps the earliest sign of ankylosing spondylitis. This movement between the iliac bones with change of posture is surely the best proof of movement in the sacroiliac joints in a normal person.

Upright Rotation

In the upright sitting position the hands are locked behind the neck, and the movements of upright rotation to the right and to the left are performed. Figure 5-28 illustrates this maneuver.

Upright rotation will only be limited by loss of function in the sacroiliac joint on the side to which the patient is turned or by pathology at the lumbosacral junction. Pathology elsewhere in the lumbar spine should not limit upright rotation. There is virtually no intervertebral rotation in the lumbar spine.

Back-Lying with Rotation

The back-lying position is adopted. The patient flops back on the examiner. The legs should remain relaxed and dangling. Back-lying in this manner exerts strain on the lumbosacral junction, and pathology here may limit this part of the examination. It is essential that the patient remain passive. In the back-lying position the trunk is rotated; Figure 5-29 shows right rotation.

As soon as the ischial tuberosity (not the buttock) on the left leaves the couch, a marked backward torsion strain is exerted on the sacroiliac joint on the right. If this position is now maintained and if pressure is exerted by the examiner's free left hand

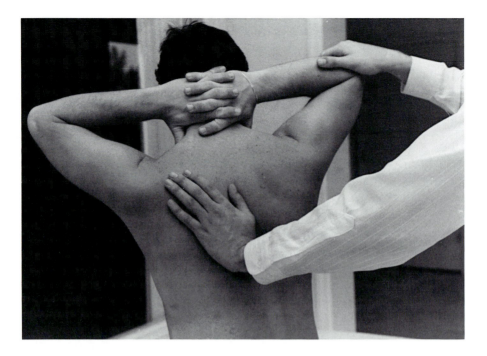

Fig. 5-28 Upright rotation to the right in the upright position. To make the movement as passive as possible the examiner's left hand pushes over the left scapula while the right hand pulls on the right elbow.

vertically over the anterior-superior spine on the left, a marked backward torsion strain is put on the sacroiliac joint on this side; this action will relieve the backward torsion strain on the right sacroiliac joint and may indeed produce a mild forward torsion strain. Put another way, back-lying with rotation of the trunk to the right exerts a marked backward torsion on the right sacroiliac joint, which is relieved by backward torsion exerted through the left sacroiliac joint. Figure 5-29 demonstrates this rather complicated maneuver.

SUPINE

The patient then lies on his or her back. In this position leg measurements are made, and a neurologic examination is undertaken.

Measurements

Muscle group atrophy is detected by measuring the circumference of the thighs and calves at 6 inches above and below the patella. To use anything but a ½-inch cloth tape is courting error. A metal tape cannot assume the contours of the leg. A thin pocket tape is easily placed around the leg obliquely without the obliquity being noticed; it can also be pulled and, unnoticed, indent the soft tissues to varying degrees.

When the thigh is measured, the patella must be pushed down to the limit of its caudal movement so that it becomes a fixed bony point from which to measure. When the calf is measured, the patella must be pushed up to the limit of its cephalad range so that it becomes a fixed bony point from which to measure. The distance of 6 inches

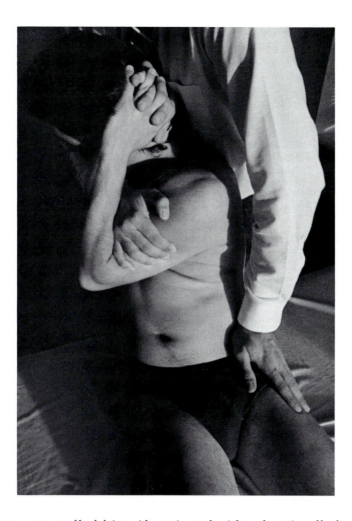

Fig. 5-29 Examining movement of back-lying with rotation to the right and exertion of backward torsion on the left sacroiliac joint. The patient is in the sitting position.

from the patella is chosen to avoid errors from atrophy of the vastus medialis or swelling in the suprapatellar pouch, both of which may be due to knee joint pathology.

The true leg lengths are then measured from beneath the anterior-superior iliac spines to below the medial tibial malleoli. When these measurements are performed the markings on the tape are ignored at first. The length of the tape is transferred from one leg to the other, and any difference in the length of the longer leg can be accurately read off by sliding the thumb at the foot end down the tape until it comes to rest below the malleolus.

Less than ½ inch discrepancy in these measurements sometimes is ignored as human error. It should always be noted, however, and may be of significance. A short leg seldom if ever causes back pain, but it may maintain back pain or provoke a recurrence. In the average back problem, the equalizing of leg lengths is not by itself a treatment for pain.

Neurologic Examination

The five leg reflexes are elicited, namely the cremasteric (labial) reflex, whose reflex arc is at the level of the first and second lumbar nerves; the patellar tendon reflex, whose arc is at the level of the third and fourth lumbar nerves; the hamstring reflex, whose arc is at the fifth lumbar level; the tendo Achilles reflex, whose arc is at the level of the first and second sacral nerves; and the plantar reflex, anomalies of which indicate pyramidal tract pathology. It should be remembered that there is an overlap in levels of these reflex arcs and that their changes do not necessarily accurately localize a level of pathology.

A sensory examination is undertaken; eliciting sensations to pin prick is sufficient. Sensory dermatomes are seldom accurate in determining levels of pathology in back conditions, but the mere presence of sensory changes is important. The main thing is to remember to prick the same area or dermatome on each leg front and back. The anal reflex will be elicited in pricking the saddle area. This reflex has its arc at the fourth and fifth sacral levels.

All these reflexes are concerned with striated voluntary muscles, having their centers within the cerebrospinal axis, and may be inhibited by voluntary effort. After spinal surgery there may be a neurologic deficit unconnected with the current problem, so that not too much reliance can be placed on doubtful neurologic signs. Even so, a useful clinical observation is that the absence of one cremasteric reflex may be the only early physical sign of a low spinal cord or high cauda equina tumor.

The feet are to be examined while the legs remain outstretched. Particular attention is paid to the resiliency of the Achilles tendons.

A patient who has a marked forefoot drop when lying supine and at rest almost always has a tendo Achilles insufficiency. This is usually associated with tightening of plantar fascia and the iliotibial band. When this happens the patient's heel cannot touch the ground at the same time as the ball of the foot without abnormal stretching of the muscles, nerves, and blood vessels in the back of the leg. This also produces abnormal tension on the back muscles and abnormal weight-bearing stresses on all the joints of the foot, the leg, and the lumbar spine (Fig. 5-30).

An uncompensated Achilles insufficiency tends to produce knee and hip extension and flattening of the lumbar lordosis. Overcompensation for the correct Achilles length (high-heeled shoes) does the reverse, and the patient stands with the knees and hips flexed, the lumbar lordosis accentuated, the thoracic kyphosis exaggerated, and the cervical lordosis increased. The head is thrust forward, which materially alters the center of gravity. This creates any or all of the symptoms of the forward head syndrome, disturbing the balance and preventing the maintenance of normal tonus of the neck muscles. This abnormal posture produces undue wear and tear in every joint in the back from the occiput to the sacrum. Muscle pain is the usual complaint, resulting from muscle spasm and fatigue. Joint dysfunction quickly ensues. Such posture predisposes to acute symptoms whenever minor trauma is inflicted on the joints. Figure 5-31 illustrates the stress effects that arise from deviations of normal resiliency in the Achilles tendon.

Correction of the full heel height must never be attempted. If it is, the remaining tendon resilience will be lost. Store-bought shoes can only have a maximum of ½ inch added to their heels without producing foot symptoms from the alteration of the slope of the soles of the shoes. In practice, added heel heights should be in the form of a wedge, which makes the maximum measurements less than ideal. The added heel should measure ½ inch posteriorly and slope forward to ¼ inch anteriorly. This actually raises the heel height only ⅜ inch. If further heel heightening is required, this can be achieved by lowering the heel on the opposite side or by adding height to the

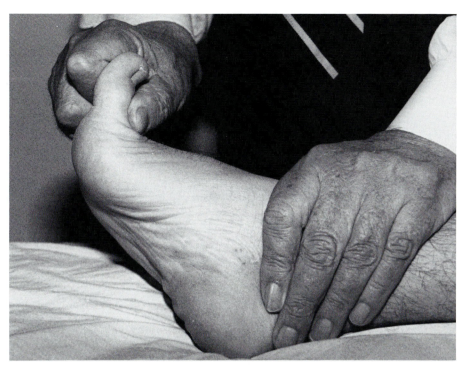

Fig. 5-30 Assessing the contour of the foot at rest, prerequisite for determining the heel height required to compensate for insufficiency of the Achilles tendon. When there is insufficiency of the Achilles tendon, the front of the foot drops markedly. The illustration shows the average drop of a normal foot.

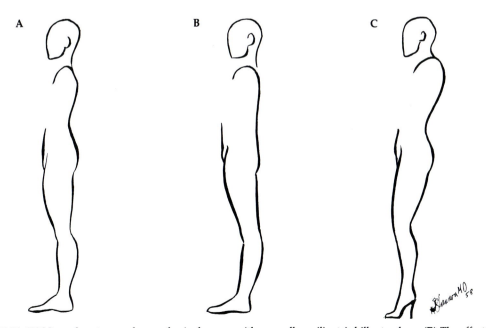

Fig. 5-31 (A) Normal posture and normal spinal curves with normally resilient Achilles tendons. (B) The effect of tendo Achilles insufficiency: extension of the knees and hips and flattening of the normal spinal curves. (C) The effect of wearing too-high heels: flexion of the knees and hips and accentuation of all the spinal curves.

sole of the shoe on the affected side as well as to the heel.

The next step is to rule out the presence of hip joint pathology, so that signs from the hip will not be confused with other signs when the hip is moved during examination of the back. This is conveniently done by rolling the outstretched leg inward and outward, these being the only hip movements that can be performed without moving other joints as well.

Straight-Leg Raising Test

The straight-leg raising test is without doubt one of the most erroneously performed and most poorly interpreted tests in common use. Limitation of straight-leg raising by pain in the low back, the back of the leg, or both is not specifically indicative of radiculitis.

Straight-leg raising may be limited and painful because of any of three conditions: (1) tight hamstring muscles, (2) sacroiliac joint pathology, and (3) radiculitis. Any of these conditions limits unilateral straight-leg raising by pain. Tightness of the hamstrings can be determined by palpation, and pain from this is usually, but not always, felt behind the knee. This should have been assessed while the patient was standing and stooping. The inability of the examiner to raise the patient's outstretched leg to 90° does not indicate an abnormality. Once hamstring muscle tightness is assessed, the examiner must differentiate between sacroiliac joint pathology and radiculitis.

At a certain angle of straight-leg raising the hamstrings pull on their origin at the ischial tuberosity. Because the opposite leg is stabilizing the other half of the pelvis, the os innominatum on the side being tested tends to be rotated backward on the sacrum through the sacroiliac joint as this muscle pull increases. At about the same angle, tension is being put on the sciatic nerve roots through pull on the sciatic trunk.

Pathology in the sacroiliac joint or radiculitis produces pain in the low back, buttock, or back of the leg. If the leg is then dropped 1 inch, both the stress on the joint and the pull on the nerve roots are relieved. With the leg stationary, the examiner *gently* dorsiflexes the foot. No painful stress is added to the sacroiliac joint, but a pull is reinstituted on the nerve roots through pull on the nerve trunk.

Exacerbation of pain on dorsiflexion of the foot is the true Lasègue's sign of radiculitis. If the pain is not reproduced by dorsiflexing the foot, sacroiliac joint pathology should be suspected.

A doubtful Lasègue sign can be checked by using Naffziger's bilateral jugular vein compression test. This test increases the pressure of the spinal fluid, which in turn increases the pressure effect of a tumor in the epidural space. It may also be checked by the head-leg test, in which tension is exerted on the low spinal roots by pulling upon them from the head end. Both legs are now raised outstretched together with the knees extended. In this, tilting tends to occur at an earlier angle of elevation than that required to move either sacroiliac joint; hence pain at an earlier angle with both legs raised together rather than separately indicates lumbosacral junction pathology.

Side-Bending of the Pelvis

The knees and hips are now flexed, with the forelegs dropping over the examiner's forearm and the hips being kept at 90°. In this position the lumbar spine is flattened, and its interlaminar joints tend to be locked except at the lumbosacral junction. When the pelvis is bent to the right, the lumbosacral facet joint on the left is opened. The lumbosacral intervertebral disc tends to be compressed on the right. Conversely, if the pelvis is bent to the left, the lumbosacral interlaminar joint is opened on the right, and the disc tends to be compressed on the left.

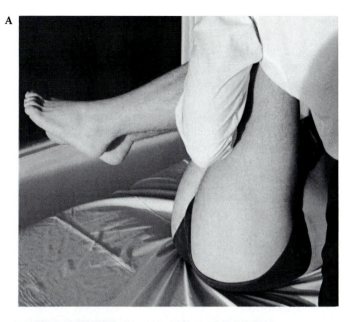

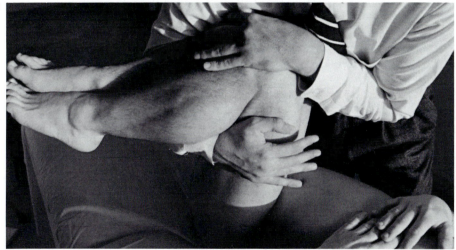

Fig. 5-32 (A) Side-bending of the pelvis to the right to open up the interlaminar articulations on the left. The lumbar spine is flattened by flexion of the hips. **(B)** Side-bending of the pelvis to the left pulls up the interlaminar articulation on the right.

Limitation of pelvic side-bending on both the right and the left by lumbosacral junction pain suggests disc pathology, bone disease, or joint disease. Figure 5-32 illustrates the movement of pelvic side-bending to the right. Some vertical downward pressure has to be put on the femoral shafts to maintain the locking of the rest of the lumbar spinal joints and to control the move-ment. Tilting at the higher facet joints in the lumbar spine can be elicited better with the patient prone.

To complete the examination of the patient in the supine position, the leg pulses must be examined because Leriche's syndrome may mimic low back pathology. Also, the abdominal examination should be performed at this time.

SIDE-LYING POSITIONS

The side-lying position is then adopted by the patient, first on one side and then on the other. The following examining movements are carried out on each side.

In the left side-lying position with the left leg fully flexed and the right leg extended, pain that is relieved by release of the left leg must have its source in the left sacroiliac joint. No pain in the static position but pain on release of the left leg must arise from a source in the lumbosacral junction. The first part of this examination is directed at further differentiation between sacroiliac joint and lumbosacral junction pathology. This is sometimes necessary when signs up to this point have been unclear. There is a circular area less than 3 inches in diameter with its center at the posterior-superior iliac spine. Around this area are five common sources of pain. Pain on palpation of any of the five indicates a different structural source of symptoms. Symptoms from these structures may mimic each other and make a diagnosis difficult.

With the patient in the left side-lying position, the left leg is drawn up onto the chest and held there by the patient. The examiner then extends the right leg, supporting the lower leg, with the knee flexed at right angles. This static position (Fig. 5-33) is maintained for a short time, and then the left leg is released (Fig. 5-34) while extension on the right leg is maintained, not increased.

Left side pain relieved by release of the left leg is coming from the left sacroiliac joint. Backward torsion strain on the sacroiliac joint, which is exerted by the fully flexed left leg pulling against the stress of the extended right leg, is relieved by release of the left leg. If the static position is painless but pain is experienced on release of the left leg, then lumbosacral junction pathology should be suspected. This is because, on release of the left leg, the tension exerted by the examiner on the

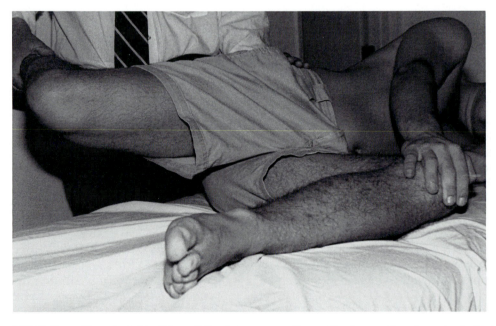

Fig. 5-33 Static position adopted in differentiating between sacroiliac and lumbosacral junction pain. In the left side-lying position, the joints on the left are considered.

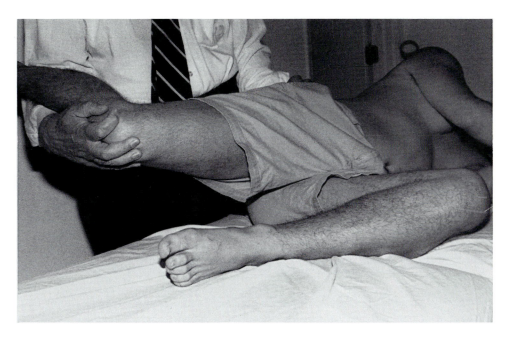

Fig. 5-34 Release of the left leg from the static position illustrated in Figure 5-33. The upper part of the right leg is not moved during this examining movement.

extended right leg causes a quick tilt of the pelvis on the fifth lumbar vertebral junction.

Iliotibial Band Resiliency

The left leg, when released, falls naturally into a flexed position of 90° at the hip and 90° at the knee. The patient is asked to hold the knee down on the table in this position. Meanwhile, the examiner lets the holding hand slide down to the ankle. The right leg is then further abducted and extended so that the iliotibial band lies over the greater trochanter of the femur (Fig. 5-35). The elevating hold of the right leg is then relaxed so that the knee may drop to the table. When the iliotibial band is pathologically tight, the knee remains suspended. When it is normally resilient, the knee falls readily toward the table top. Usually there is diffuse fibrositic tenderness in a tight iliotibial band.

Forward Torsion of the Ilium on the Sacrum

The position of the patient's legs is then reversed, the right leg dropping in front of the lower leg which remains as straight as possible. The fingers of the examiner's left hand hold the patient's right wrist. If this is not relaxed, then the patient is not relaxed, and normal play movements cannot safely be obtained.

The heel of the right hand is then placed just behind the anterior-superior iliac spine in the fossa between the sartorius in the front and the tensor fascia lata behind. The pelvis is obliqued forward. The trunk is rotated backward by the examiner's pulling on the chest wall with the left forearm and elbow. This locks all facet joints. The play movement is achieved by exerting a downward and somewhat oblique thrust over the anterior third of the patient's iliac crest directed caudally, using the heel of the hand. Figure 5-36 illustrates this maneuver.

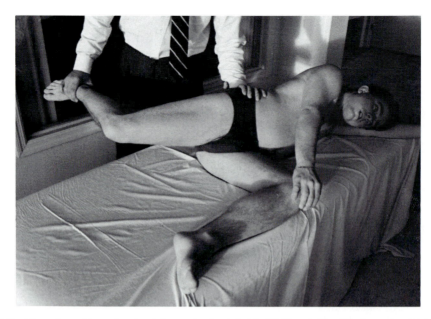

Fig. 5-35 Position adopted in testing for tightness in the right iliotibial band. The right knee should drop toward the table resiliently.

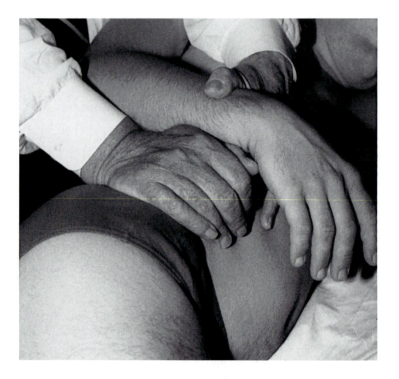

Fig. 5-36 Position adopted for performing the forward torsion examination of the right sacroiliac joint in the left side-lying position.

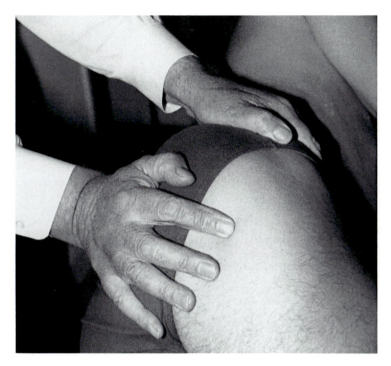

Fig. 5-37 Position adopted for performing the backward torsion examination of the right sacroiliac joint in the left side-lying position.

Backward Torsion of the Ilium on the Sacrum

Backward torsion on the right sacroiliac joint is produced by pulling backward on the patient's anterior-superior iliac spine with the left hand and pushing forward over the ischial tuberosity with the right hand in the arc of a circle. Figure 5-37 illustrates this examining movement.

PRONE

The patient now assumes the face-down or prone position. The distance between the posterior-superior iliac spines is measured for the second time and compared with the measurement made in the upright sitting position. In the absence of sacroiliac joint disease, there should be a spread of these spines of up to ¼ to ¾ inch.

Skin Rolling

The next examining procedure is skin rolling up the spine. Skin rolling is difficult to describe and to illustrate. It is a smooth rolling of the skin over the spinous processes of the vertebrae by the fingers over the advancing thumbs. Figure 5-38 shows how the skin is picked up preparatory to rolling it up the back. Skin rolling is performed over the vertebrae and then over each paravertebral area.

Fibrositic infiltration, trigger points, and other muscular pathologic states are demonstrated by tightness and acute tenderness. There will be tightness and

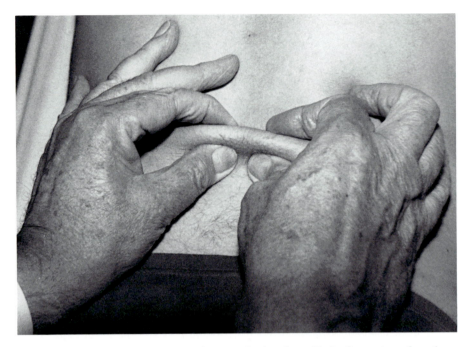

Fig. 5-38 Manner in which the skin is picked up between the thumbs and index fingers to perform the maneuver of skin rolling.

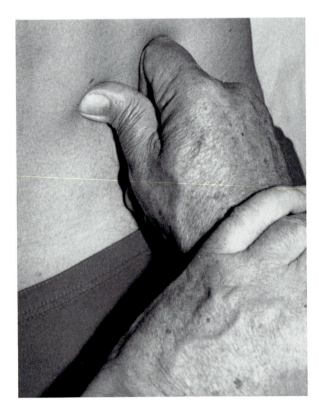

Fig. 5-39 Application of direct pressure over a specific vertebra. The spinous process is cradled between the thumb and the flexed index finger to avoid unnatural rotation of the vertebra during the thrusting movement.

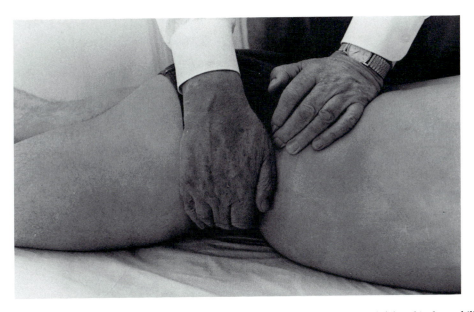

Fig. 5-40 Position adopted to move an individual facet joint in the lumbar spine. The left hand is the mobilizing hand. At each higher level, the right hand takes up more slack. The examiner's mobilizing left hand should not be over the vertebral transverse process, which may easily break off.

tenderness at whatever level pathologic change exists. In joint dysfunction, skin rolling elicits tenderness at one intervertebral junction and at the same level when the skin is rolled paravertebrally on the painful side. On the opposite side there may be little if any tenderness and tightness. The examiner may find a localized area of tightness and tenderness that is inconsistent with any structure of the musculoskeletal system of the back. In such a case the organ next deep from the skin should be suspected as the source of pain because of a pathologic state in it.

Direct Vertical Thrust

The level of probable bone, joint, or disc pathology as determined by the skin rolling test is confirmed by a direct thrust over each individual vertebra. To avoid an abnormal rotatory movement during this procedure, the thrust is achieved by flexing the forefinger to place the horizontal middle phalanx on one side of the spinous process and the hyperextended terminal phalanx of the thumb on the other side of the spinous process (Fig. 5-39). This cradles the spinous process between the thumb and forefinger, and the downward thrust is equal over the lateral masses on each side. This movement is performed over each lumbar vertebra.

Should there still be some doubt as to the level of pathology, each facet joint can be tested for sagittal joint play movement. To examine the right facet joints, the examiner stands on the left side of the patient. The pisiform of the left hand is placed over the mamillary process of the facet joint to be examined. While the mamillary process is held down, the right hand lifts the anterior-superior iliac spine until it appears that the facet is engaging under the left hand. The left hand takes up any further slack and then thrusts directly toward the floor to accomplish the less than ⅛ inch play movement. Figure 5-40 illustrates the position adopted for this movement.

PALPATION

Finally there are 14 local areas (7 on each side) in which tenderness on palpation is constant in certain conditions. There are 5 areas on each side of the back to be examined, 1 in each buttock, and 1 in the back of each thigh.

The 7 areas in each side are as follows:

1. One fingerbreadth medial to the posterior-superior iliac spine is the most superficial posterior ligament of the sacroiliac joint.
2. One fingerbreadth lateral to the posterior-superior iliac spine is the puny part of the gluteal muscle origin, which may be torn by minor trauma. Tenderness here suggests the presence of a muscle tear.
3. One fingerbreadth above the posterior-superior iliac spine is the musculotendinous junction of the sacrospinalis muscles. Muscle fiber tears frequently occur at this junction with minor lifting trauma. Tenderness here suggests muscle fiber tears.
4. One fingerbreadth above and medial to the posterior-superior iliac spine is the area over the interlaminar facet joint, where tenderness may occur if dysfunction is present.
5. One fingerbreadth medial and inferior to area 4 above is the area where local tenderness may occur from disc pathology.
6. Halfway between the ischial tuberosity of the femur the sciatic nerve emerges from beneath the piriformis muscle. This suggests either spasm of the muscle or radicular pathology.
7. Tenderness on palpating across the sciatic trunk in the back of the thigh indicates neuritis.

RECTAL AND PELVIC EXAMINATIONS

The low back examination is then completed by a rectal and, if appropriate, a pelvic examination. The lower ligaments of the sacroiliac joints can be palpated, and in some people the anterior aspect of the lumbosacral junction can be felt. The whole of the sacrum should be palpated anteriorly. The piriformis muscle can be palpated. The uterus and its cervix can be assessed. The ovaries and salpinges can be appraised. The prostate is also examined.

III. Normal Joint Play in the Synovial Joints of the Wrists and Hands

THE FINGERS

Metacarpophalangeal and Interphalangeal Joints

The range of joint play in the metacarpophalangeal joints and in the interphalangeal joints is the same in movement but differs in extent. The movements of joint play are long axis extension, anteroposterior tilt, side tilt medially and laterally, and rotation. Because the metacarpophalangeal joint of the index finger is the most easily handled joint in the body and is easily visualized radiographically, it is used to illustrate the extent of movement achieved on examination. Reference to the illustrations makes it clear that the extent of the movements of joint play is small compared to the extent of the voluntary movements that are dependent upon them. The fact that the movements are small does not mean that their importance is not great. Because they are small, however, it is of vital importance that the examination is performed precisely.

Long Axis Extension

The examiner holds the head of the metacarpal bone between the thumb and index finger and then grasps the shaft of the proximal phalanx in a golf club grip. The examiner then pulls the base of the phalanx away from the head of the metacarpal bone. It should be noted clinically that, on completion of long axis extension, none of the soft tissue structures is stretched; only the normal slack in them is taken up.

Figure 5-41 illustrates the position adopted to perform this joint play movement of long axis extension. Figure 5-42 demonstrates radiographically the relationship of the same two bones before the movement (ie, with the joint at rest), and Figure 5-43 demonstrates radiographically the relationship of the articular surfaces of the bones at the end of the movement of long axis extension. One should note the wide separation of the bones at the completion of long axis extension (Fig. 5-43) compared to their relative positions at rest (Fig. 5-42). The radial relationship of subchondral bone surfaces at rest should be noticed because this relationship is maintained throughout all voluntary movements, as shown in Figure 5-42. It differs widely in the performance of joint play movements.

Anteroposterior Tilt

The examiner maintains the grip upon the head of the metacarpal bone and places the tip of the thumb of the other hand just distal to the base of the phalanx posteriorly and the tip of the index finger just distal to the base of the phalanx anteriorly. By applying pressure with the thumb and the index finger alternately, the examiner then tilts the base of the phalanx alternately backward and forward, using either the thumb or the index finger as a fulcrum. Thus the metacarpophalangeal joint is tilted open, first posteriorly and then anteriorly. The joint is held in about 10° of flexion. Figure 5-44 shows the position adopted to elicit the tilt; Figure 5-45 shows the anterior tilt.

One should observe that these are not shearing movements but pure tilting movements that open up the joint space anteriorly and posteriorly, again without stretching any of the supporting soft tissues. Figure 5-46 shows radiographically the relationship of the articular surfaces of

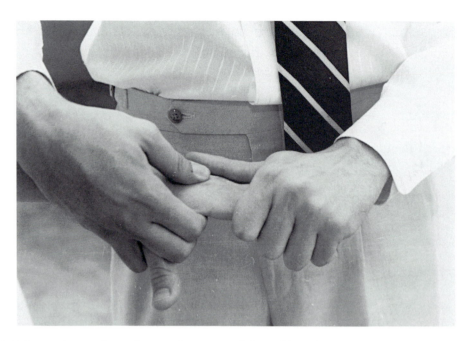

Fig. 5-41 Long axis extension at the second metacarpophalangeal joint demonstrating the golf club grip by the examiner's mobilizing right hand and stabilization of the head of the metacarpal bone by the left hand.

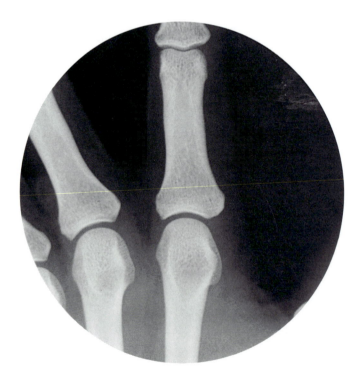

Fig. 5-42 Radiograph of the metacarpophalangeal joint of the index finger at rest. *Source*: Reprinted from *Back Pain: Diagnosis and Treatment Using Manipulative Techniques* (p 19) by John Mennell with permission of Little, Brown and Company, © 1960.

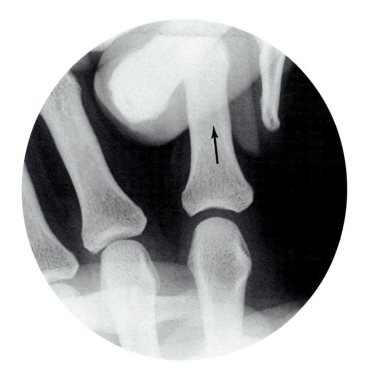

Fig. 5-43 Radiograph of the metacarpophalangeal joint of the index finger at the limit of long axis extension. The relationship of the articulating surfaces of the bones should be compared to their relationship with the joint at rest. *Source*: Reprinted from *Back Pain: Diagnosis and Treatment Using Manipulative Techniques* (p 19) by John Mennell with permission of Little, Brown and Company, © 1960.

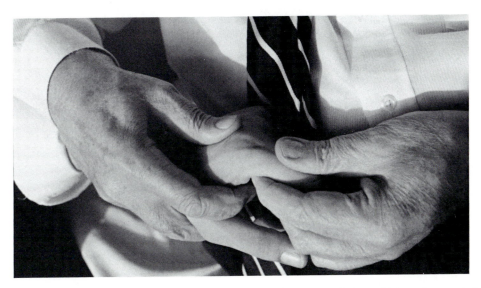

Fig. 5-44 Position adopted to elicit the backward tilt of the second metacarpophalangeal joint at the completion of the movement, which is almost entirely performed by use of the profundus muscle of the examiner's left index finger.

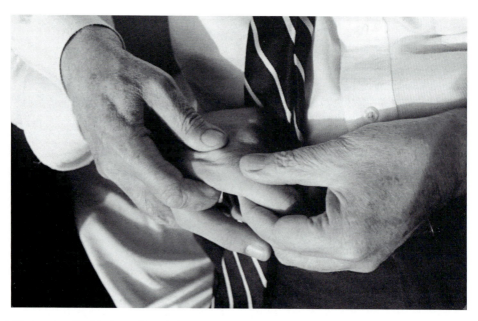

Fig. 5-45 Anterior tilt of the base of the phalanx on the head of the second metacarpal bone. The examiner uses the thumb of the left hand as the mobilizing unit. The tilt must not be a glide.

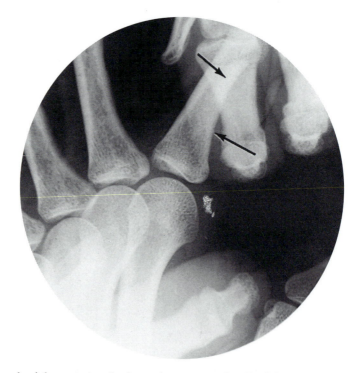

Fig. 5-46 Radiograph of the posterior tilt phase of anteroposterior tilt of the metacarpophalangeal joint. The difference between the radial relationship of the articulating surfaces of the bones in this position and their relationship in flexion should be noted. *Source*: Reprinted from *Back Pain: Diagnosis and Treatment Using Manipulative Techniques* (p 20) by John Mennell with permission of Little, Brown and Company, © 1960.

the bones at the limit of the posterior phase of this movement, and Figure 5-47 shows their relationship at the limit of the anterior phase of this movement.

The position of the base of the phalanx in relation to the head of the metacarpal bone should be noted in the voluntary movement of flexion (Fig. 5-48) and compared with the relative positions when the joint space is tilted open medially (Figs. 5-49 and 5-50) and with the joint in abduction (Fig. 5-51).

Side Tilt Medially and Laterally

The examiner maintains the grip on the head of the metacarpal bone and places the thumb and index finger of the other hand on the medial and lateral sides of the prox-

imal phalanx, respectively, just distal to its base. The thumb is used as a pivot, and the metacarpophalangeal joint is tilted open medially by pressure exerted through the tip of the index finger. Then the tip of the index finger is used as a pivot, and the metacarpophalangeal joint is tilted open laterally by pressure exerted through the thumb. Figure 5-49 illustrates the position adopted to open up the lateral aspect of the joint.

Rotation

The examiner maintains the grip on the head of the metacarpal bone and flexes the proximal and distal ends of the proximal phalanx between the thumb and index and middle fingers. The examiner places the

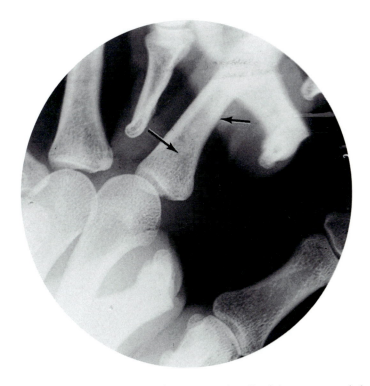

Fig. 5-47 Radiograph of the anterior tilt phase of anteroposterior tilt of the metacarpophalangeal joint. The difference between the radial relationship of the articulating surfaces of the bones in this position and their relationship in flexion should be noted. *Source*: Reprinted from *Back Pain: Diagnosis and Treatment Using Manipulative Techniques* (p 20) by John Mennell with permission of Little, Brown and Company, © 1960.

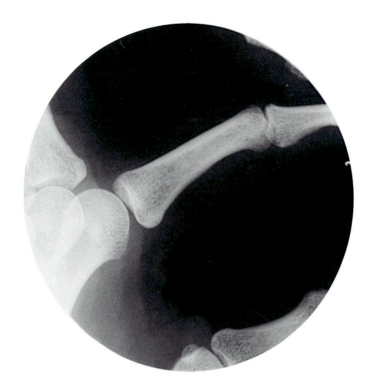

Fig. 5-48 Radiograph of the metacarpophalangeal joint of the index finger in flexion. Note that the radial relationship of the bones is the same as when the finger is at rest. *Source*: Reprinted from *Back Pain: Diagnosis and Treatment Using Manipulative Techniques* (p 19) by John Mennell with permission of Little, Brown and Company, © 1960.

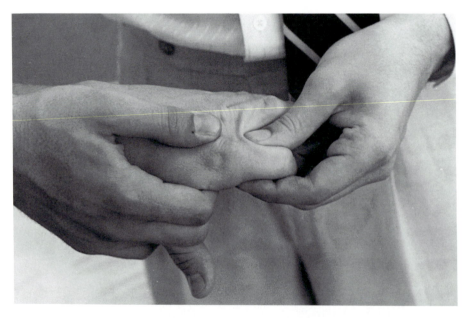

Fig. 5-49 Lateral tilt opening up the lateral aspect of a metacarpophalangeal joint. Note that the examiner's left thumb is being used as a pivot while the index finger tilts the base of the phalanx away from the metacarpal bone.

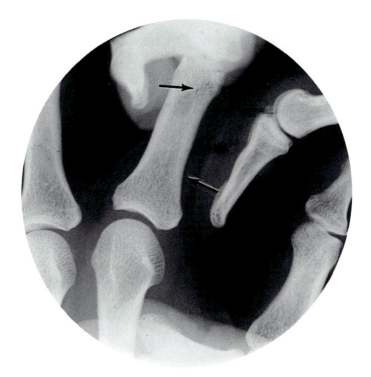

Fig. 5-50 Radiograph of the metacarpophalangeal joint side-tilted open medially. The radial relationship of the articulating surfaces of the bones in this position and their relationship in abduction (Fig. 5-51) and at rest (Fig. 5-42) should be noted. *Source*: Reprinted from *Back Pain: Diagnosis and Treatment Using Manipulative Techniques* (p 20) by John Mennell with permission of Little, Brown and Company, © 1960.

fourth finger on the other side of the subject's middle phalanx, thus crooking the subject's finger between the examining fingers. The examiner then rotates the proximal phalanx clockwise and counterclockwise in its long axis, the base of this phalanx thus rotating upon the head of the metacarpal bone. Figure 5-52 illustrates the position adopted to elicit this movement.

In examining for this movement at a distal interphalangeal joint, there is no way of crooking the subject's finger to produce leverage. In the distal interphalangeal joint the movement has to be elicited by simple rotation in the long axis, maintaining the head of the middle phalanx in the stable position.

Figure 5-53 illustrates the position of the base of the phalanx in relation to the head

of the metacarpal bone at the completion of counterclockwise rotation in the movement of joint play. The extent of the movement of the base of the phalanx on the head of the metacarpal bone is best appreciated when their positions are compared to those shown in any of the radiographs in this chapter.

THE HAND

The Distal Intermetacarpal Joints

The movements of joint play between the heads of each metacarpal bone are anteroposterior glide and rotation. Of course, the

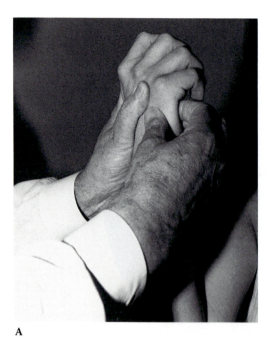

A

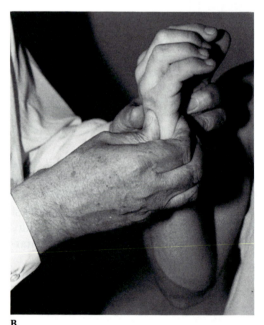

B

Fig. 5-54 (A) Completion of the posterior (dorsal) phase of anteroposterior glide of the head of the fifth metacarpal bone on the head of the fourth. The head of the fourth is stabilized by the examiner's right hand. **(B)** Completion of the anterior (volar) phase of anteroposterior glide of the head of the fifth metacarpal bone on that of the fourth. The head of the fourth metacarpal bone is being stabilized.

Anteroposterior Glide

With the subject's elbow flexed and the forearm in the neutral position, the examiner stands facing the dorsum of the hand. The examiner grasps the neck of the fourth metacarpal bone between the fingers and thumb of the right hand and the neck of the fifth metacarpal bone between the thumb and index finger of the left hand, moving the fifth metacarpal bone forward and backward on the stabilized head of the fourth metacarpal bone. The head of the fourth metacarpal bone is moved in a similar way on the stabilized head of the third metacarpal bone. Figure 5-54A shows the completion of the dorsal movement, and Figure 5-54B shows the completion of the volar movement. The examiner reverses the role of the hands when moving the head of the second metacarpal bone forward and backward on the stabilized head of the third metacarpal bone.

Rotation

The examiner stabilizes the fourth metacarpal bone by holding its neck between the thumb and index finger of the right hand. The examiner then grasps the neck of the fifth metacarpal bone between the thumb and index finger of the left hand and, with a shoulder swing, rotates the head of the fifth metacarpal bone, first clockwise and then counterclockwise.

Figure 5-55A illustrates the extreme of clockwise rotation, and Figure 5-55B illustrates the extreme of counterclockwise rotation. The head of the fourth metacarpal bone is moved in a similar way on the stabilized head of the third metacarpal bone. The role of the examiner's hands is reversed to rotate in both directions the head of the second metacarpal bone on the stabilized head of the third metacarpal bone.

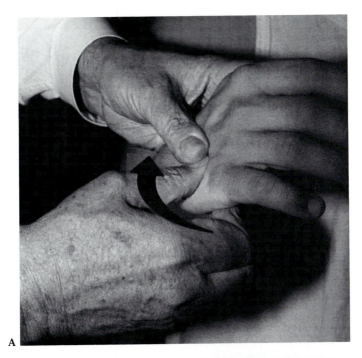

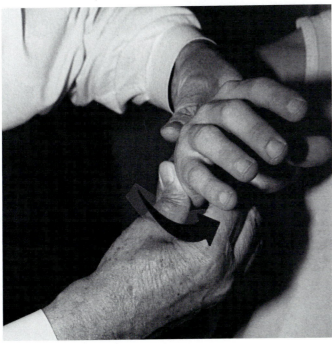

Fig. 5-55 (**A**) Anterior (clockwise) rotation of the head of the fifth metacarpal bone on that of the fourth. The head of the fourth metacarpal bone is being stabilized. Compare the position of the examiner's left thumb and index finger (the mobilizing hand) with that used when performing the anteroposterior glide, as illustrated in Figures 5-7 and 5-12. (**B**) Posterior (counterclockwise) rotation of the head of the fifth metacarpal bone on that of the fourth. The head of the fourth metacarpal bone is being stabilized.

The Carpometacarpal Joints

It is almost impossible to demonstrate the play of metacarpal bones on the distal row of carpal bones. Loss of function in these joints cannot be demonstrated specifically except that, when the distal row of carpal bones is tilted backward on the proximal row, the fingers do not spread and extend as they should. This results from loss of play. Such movement as takes place at the carpometacarpal joints is purely involuntary, and its presence or absence must be observed while examination for the movements at the midcarpal joint is being undertaken.

THE WRIST

When it is remembered that there are 16 synovial joints that make up the wrist, it will be realized that it is rather ingenuous to talk of a painful wrist. The eight carpal bones of the wrist are involved in two major functional joints, however, which makes our discussion of this much simpler. Figure 5-56 is a schematic illustration showing these two major composite joints at the wrist and the joints that control supination and pronation. For clinical purposes, the wrist may be divided into three major clinical areas: the midcarpal joint, the radiocarpal joints, and the ulnomeniscocarpal

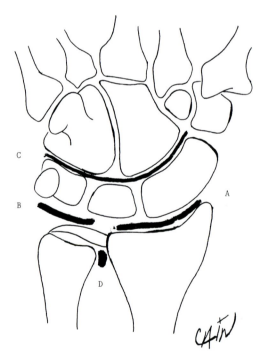

Fig. 5-56 Diagrammatic illustration of the carpal bones showing the four main composite joints at the wrist. For the most part, extension occurs at the midcarpal joint (C), whereas for the most part flexion occurs at the radioulnocarpal joint (A). (B) is the ulnomeniscocarpal joint, which for the most part controls supination. (D) is the radioulnar joint, which for the most part controls pronation.

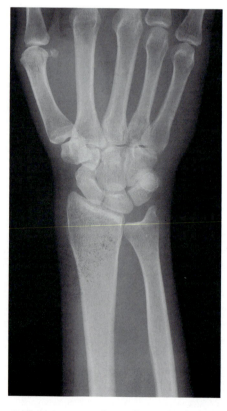

Fig. 5-57 Anteroposterior radiograph of a normal wrist. The major clinical joints are indicated and designated in Figure 5-56 as follows: (A) radiocarpal joint, (B) ulnomeniscocarpal joint, and (C) midcarpal joint.

joint. Figure 5-57, an anteroposterior radiographic view of a normal left wrist, shows the relationship of the bones of the carpus to each other and to the lower ends of the radius and ulna proximally and to the bases of the metacarpal bones distally. These relationships should be kept in mind and compared with those at the completion of the normal joint play movements described and illustrated later.

Normal Voluntary Movements

For the most part, extension at the wrist takes place at the midcarpal joint. This is made up of the articular surfaces of the navicular and lunate bones proximally, and the articulate surfaces of the capitate and hamate bones distally. Figure 5-58 is a lateral radiographic view of a normal wrist in extension. It clearly shows that this movement occurs for the most part at the midcarpal joints. Figure 5-59 shows flexion in a normal wrist for comparison.

For the most part, flexion takes place at the radiocarpal joint, which is made up of the articular surface of the lower end of the radius and the articular surfaces of the navicular and lunate bones. The ulnomeniscocarpal (ulnomeniscotriquetral) joint is largely concerned with the function of supination of the forearm. There is one other joint at the wrist that is often overlooked: the inferior radioulnar joint. This is involved in the movement of pronation.

Thus when a patient presents with inability to flex the wrist or complains of pain while performing this movement, one's attention should be focused on the radiocarpal joint. If the patient presents with an inability to extend the wrist or complains of pain while attempting to perform this movement, one's attention should be focused on the midcarpal joint. Finally, if the presenting complaint is inability to supinate the forearm or pain on attempting

this movement, one's attention should be directed at the ulnomeniscocarpal joint. If the presenting complaint is inability to pronate the forearm or pain on attempting this movement, one's attention should be directed at the distal radioulnar joint.

For illustration of the joint play movements in these joints of the wrist, the model's left wrist is being examined in most cases.

The Midcarpal Joint

The movements of joint play at this joint are long axis extension, anteroposterior glide, and backward tilt of the distal carpal bones on the proximal carpal bones.

Long Axis Extension

With the subject's elbow flexed at a right angle and the forearm in the neutral position between supination and pronation, the examiner places the right hand anteriorly over the condylar region of the subject's humerus at the elbow. The examiner then grasps the wrist area with the left hand, the thumb being just distal to the radial styloid process and the index finger just distal to the ulnar styloid process (where, it will be noted, there are natural indentations that prevent the thumb and finger from slipping down the hand when a pull is exerted). Figure 5-60 illustrates the position adopted to elicit this movement. The examiner exerts traction with the left hand by using a rotatory body swing and stabilizes the subject's forearm by countertraction, pressure being applied with the right hand at the lower end of the subject's upper arm.

Anteroposterior Glide

With the subject's arm flexed at the elbow and the forearm in the neutral posi-

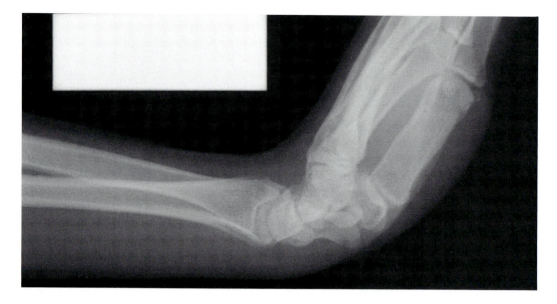

Fig. 5-58 Lateral radiograph of the normal wrist at the completion of the normal voluntary movement of extension. Note that the movement largely occurs at the midcarpal joint. Comparison should be made with Figure 5-59, which shows the wrist in flexion.

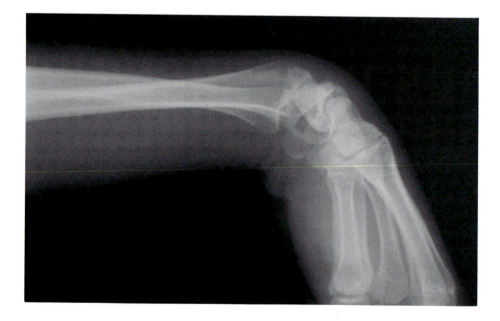

Fig. 5-59 Lateral radiograph of a normal wrist at the completion of the normal voluntary movement of flexion. Note that the movement largely occurs at the radiocarpal joint. Comparison should be made with Figure 5-58, which shows the wrist in extension.

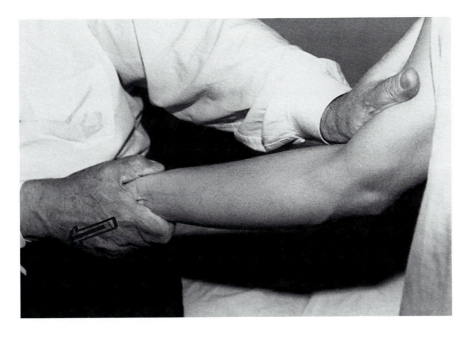

Fig. 5-60 Position adopted to produce long axis extension at the midcarpal joint. Arrow shows direction of pull used to execute this movement.

tion, the examiner grasps the subject's wrist with the right hand so that the thumb and forefinger are placed over the proximal row of carpal bones dorsally. The examiner's wrist is extended so that the metacarpophalangeal joints rest over the long axis of the lower end of the radius. The left hand, also dorsiflexed, grasps the subject's hand so that the thumb and forefinger are placed over the distal row of carpal bones and the metacarpophalangeal line is also in the long axis of the subject's radius. The subject's wrist is flexed. The examiner's right hand stabilizes the proximal row of carpal bones, and the left hand thrusts forward in such a way that the line of force approximates the index finger of the examiner's left hand toward the index finger of the right hand at an angle of about 45°. Figure 5-61 illustrates the position adopted to elicit this movement.

Figure 5-62 is a lateral radiographic view of the midcarpal joint at completion of the anterior phase of the anteroposterior glide joint play movement. The extent of the movement would be greater had it been technically possible to make the exposure with the forearm held in the neutral position instead of in a considerable degree of pronation. However, if one compares this picture with Figure 5-57 (a lateral view of the normal wrist at rest), there can be no doubt that the normal joint play movement of anteroposterior glide occurs at the midcarpal joint.

This achieves the anterior phase of anteroposterior glide; the posterior phase is achieved when the thrust is released and rebound into the neutral position occurs. It should be noted that anteroposterior glide cannot be demonstrated with the subject's forearm in full supination or full pronation.

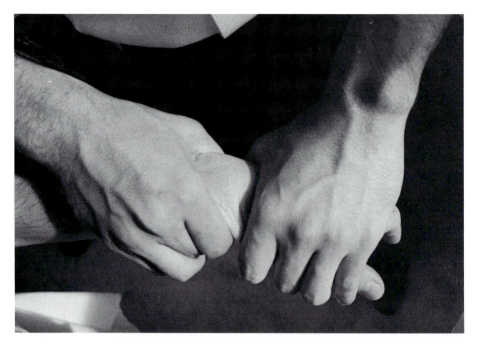

Fig. 5-61 Position adopted to elicit anteroposterior movement at the midcarpal joint. Note that the examiner's wrists are dorsiflexed so that the thrusting force of the mobilizing left hand is parallel to the joint line.

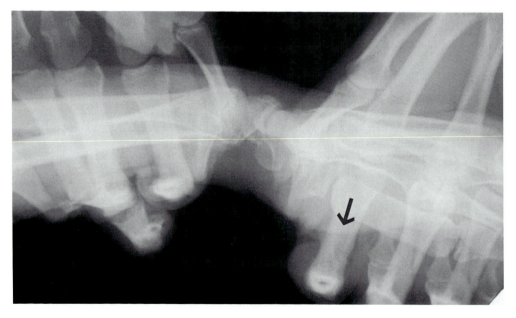

Fig. 5-62 The midcarpal joint at the completion of the anterior phase of the joint play movement of anteroposterior glide. The arrow at the right shows the direction of thrust.

Backward Tilt of the Capitate on the Lunate and Navicular

With the subject's arm flexed at the elbow and the forearm held in the vertical and neutral position, the examiner places the thenar eminence of the right hand on the volar aspect of the subject's proximal row of carpal bones and the thenar eminence of the left hand on the dorsal aspect of the subject's distal row of carpal bones, clasping the fingers around the radial aspect of the subject's wrist. The examiner dorsiflexes the wrists so that the long axis of the radii are directed at right angles to the subject's carpus. The examiner then squeezes the hands together, thrusting together the thenar eminences in the long axis of the radii. This movement tilts the subject's distal row of carpal bones backward upon the proximal row of carpal bones, particularly the capitate on the navicula and lunate, tilting the anterior aspect of the midcarpal joint open. The capitate tilts backward.

Figure 5-63 illustrates the position adopted to achieve this movement. The extension and spread of the subject's fingers should be noted because these are the only demonstrable criteria that the midcarpal joint movement has been properly accomplished. Figure 5-64 shows tracings taken from a double exposure; Figure 5-64A shows the position adopted to perform the procedure, and Figure 5-64B shows the position of the fingers at the completion of the movement.

Intercarpal Joints

There is, of course, a range of movement between each carpal bone. This cannot be readily appreciated on clinical examination unless there has been a traumatic subluxation of one of the bones upon another. This most commonly happens in the wrist when the lunate bone subluxes backward on its adjacent carpal bones. The range of specific

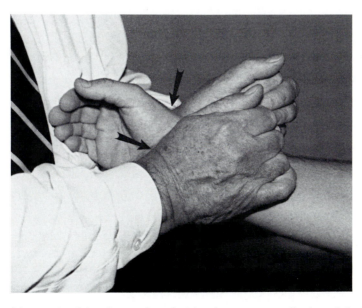

Fig. 5-63 Position of the examiner's hands to perform the joint play movement of backward tilt of the distal carpal bones on the proximal carpal bones. The performance of this movement depends upon the accurate placement of the examiner's thenar eminences over the correct bones.

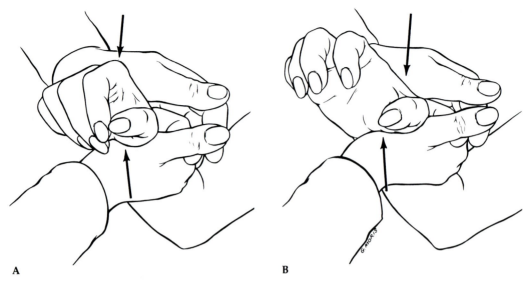

A   B

Fig. 5-64 (A) Tracing illustrating the position of the examiner's hands and the subject's right hand to produce the joint play movement of backward tilt of the distal carpal bones on the proximal carpal bones. **(B)** Tracing illustrating the position of the examiner's hands and the subject's right hand at the completion of the joint play movement of backward tilt of the distal carpal bones on the proximal carpal bones. Note the extension and spreading of the subject's fingers, which take place only when this joint play movement is elicited correctly.

involuntary movement is probably such that each bone can just move forward and backward upon its neighboring bones.

The Radiocarpal Joint

The radiocarpal joint is the composite joint between the distal end of the radius and the navicular and lunate bones. The movements of joint play at this joint are long axis extension, backward tilt of the navicular and lunate bones on the lower end of the radius, and side tilt of the navicula on the radius.

Long Axis Extension

Long axis extension at this joint is achieved in exactly the same manner as long axis extension at the midcarpal joint. With the subject's elbow fixed at a right angle and the forearm in midposition, the examiner places the right hand anteriorly over the condylar region of the subject's

humerus at the elbow. The examiner then grasps the wrist area with the left hand, the thumb being just distal to the radial styloid process (where, it will be noted, there is a natural indentation that prevents the thumb and finger from slipping down the hand when a pull is exerted). The examiner exerts traction with the left hand by using a rotatory body swing while stabilizing the forearm by countertraction, applying pressure with the right hand at the subject's elbow.

Backward Tilt of the Navicular and
Lunate Bones on the Radius

The examiner stands facing the subject with the latter's arm flexed at the elbow and the forearm pronated. The examiner places the right thumb over the dorsal aspect of the navicula, the thumb being in the long axis of the subject's radius, and places the left thumb over the lunate, the thumb again being in the long axis of the subject's

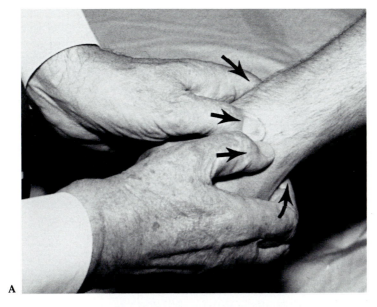

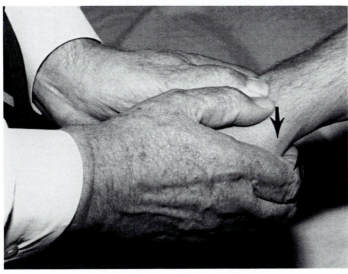

Fig. 5-65 **(A)** Position of the examiner's hands to elicit the backward tilt of the navicular and lunate bones upon the lower end of the radius. The examiner's right thumb and index finger grasp the navicula; the examiner's left thumb and index finger grasp the lunate. **(B)** Side-on view of the position illustrated in Fig. 5-65A. The examiner is grasping the subject's navicular and lunate bones before eliciting their backward tilt upon the lower end of the radius.

radius. The examiner then crooks the index fingers around the wrist so that they lie at right angles to the thumbs but on the volar surface; their tips are placed over the navicula and the lunate in such a manner that the examiner is grasping the navicula with the right hand and the lunate with the left hand. Figure 5-65 illustrates the position adopted to perform the movement and the position at the completed movement.

The navicula and the lunate are gently flexed forward on the lower end of the radius as the forearm is being gently raised by the examiner's slightly increasing flexion at the elbow. The forearm is then whipped downward toward the floor by sudden ulnar deviation of the examiner's wrists, the movement being arrested in such a way that, momentarily, the navicula and lunate are tilted backward on the lower end of the radius, which tilts the radiocarpal joint open at its volar aspect.

Side Tilt of the Navicula on the Radius

The examiner grasps the lower end of the radius and ulna between the thumb and index finger of the right hand and the proximal row of carpal bones between the thumb and index finger of the left hand, holding the subject's arm in the neutral position and flexed at the elbow. Using the thumbs as a pivot, the examiner stabilizes the lower end of the forearm bones with the right hand and, by ulnar deviation of the left wrist, tilts the navicula away from the lower end of the radius. The position adopted to elicit this movement is shown in Figure 5-66. Figure 5-67 is a radiograph taken at the completion of the

joint play movement of side tilt of the navicula on the lower end of the radius. The extent of this movement may be seen if one compares the relationship of these two bones in Figure 5-67 with that when they are at rest.

The Ulnomeniscotriquetral Joint

The movements of joint play at the ulnomeniscocarpal (ulnomeniscotriquetral) joint are anteroposterior glide and side tilt. Although long axis extension occurs at this joint and is performed as illustrated for the same play movement at the radiocarpal joint, it is of little clinical importance because of the meniscus separating the articular surfaces of the ulna and the triquetrum.

Anteroposterior Glide

With the subject's arm flexed at the elbow and the forearm held in the vertical and neutral position, the examiner holds the radial half of the subject's hand in the right hand. The examiner then places the

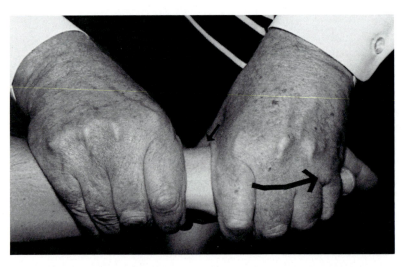

Fig. 5-66 Joint play movement of side tilt of the navicula away from the radius. The examiner's right hand stabilizes the lower end of the radius. By using both thumbs as a pivot, the examiner tilts the navicula away from the lower end of the radius by turning the left hand into ulnar deviation.

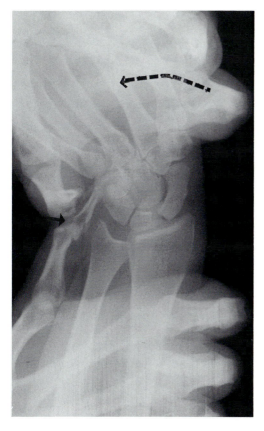

Fig. 5-67 Radiograph showing the completion of the joint play movement of side tilt of the navicula away from the radius.

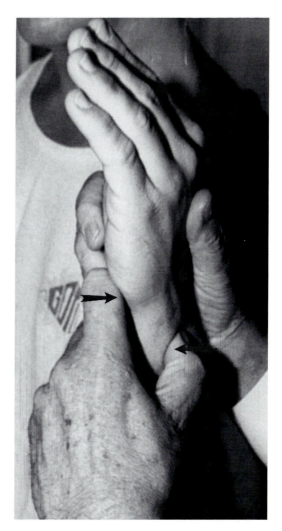

Fig. 5-68 Position at the completion of anteroposterior glide of the ulna on the triquetrum (between which lies a meniscus) in its anterior phase. The posterior phase is achieved on rebound from this position. Note that the examiner's right hand merely stabilizes the subject's left hand and arm. The movement by the examiner is achieved by pinching together the left thumb and forefinger in parallel.

left thumb over the posterior aspect of the neck of the lower end of the ulna, the thumb being at right angles to the long axis of the ulna. The examiner next crooks the left index finger and places its proximal interphalangeal joint over the pisiform bone on the volar aspect of the subject's wrist. The examiner then pinches the left thumb and index finger together, thereby carrying the lower end of the subject's ulna forward on the triquetrum as the triquetrum moves backward on the lower end of the ulna and the meniscus that lies between them. Figure 5-68 illustrates the position adopted to elicit the movement,

the photograph being taken at the completion of it. Figure 5-69 should be compared with Figure 5-62 for a better appreciation of the nature of the joint play movement of anteroposterior glide at the midcarpal joint.

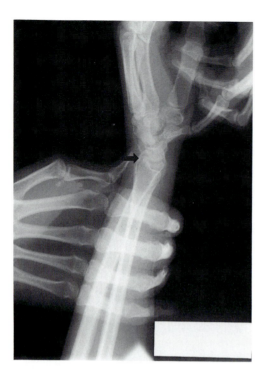

Fig. 5-69 Joint play between the lower end of the ulna and the triquetral bone (ulnomeniscotriquetral joint) toward the completion of the joint play movement of anterior glide.

Side Tilt of the Triquetrum on the Ulna

The examiner grasps the lower ends of the radius and ulna between the thumb and index finger of the right hand and the proximal row of carpal bones between the thumb and index finger of the left hand, holding the subject's arm in the neutral position and flexed at the elbow. Using the index fingers as a pivot, the examiner stabilizes the lower end of the forearm bones with the right hand and tilts the subject's hand into radial deviation with the left hand. Figure 5-70 demonstrates the position adopted to elicit this movement.

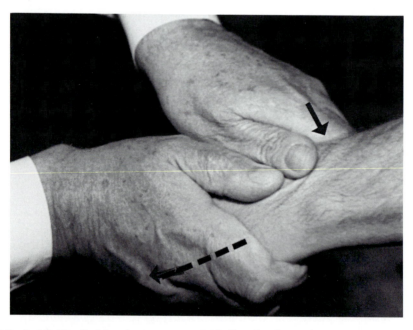

Fig. 5-70 Method of eliciting the joint play movement of side tilt at the ulnomeniscotriquetral joint. The examiner uses the index finger of the left hand as a pivot at the radiocarpal joint and pulls the subject's hand into radial deviation with the right hand, thus tilting the triquetrum away from the lower end of the ulna and the meniscus upon which it rests.

The Inferior Radioulnar Joint

The movements of joint play at this joint are anteroposterior glide and rotation of the lower end of the ulna on the radius.

Anteroposterior Glide

With the subject's arm flexed at the elbow and the forearm held in the vertical and neutral position, the examiner places the right thumb posteriorly over the neck of the lower end of the ulna, the thumb being at right angles to the long axis of the radius. The tip of the right index finger is placed on the anterior surface at the lower end of the ulna. The examiner stabilizes the lower end of the radius with the right hand and alternately pushes the lower end of the ulna forward and backward upon it. Figure 5-71 illustrates the position adopted to elicit this movement.

Rotation

Using the same examining position as described for eliciting the joint play movement of anteroposterior glide at this joint, the examiner stabilizes the lower end of the radius with the right hand and rotates the lower end of the subject's ulna on its own axis by using an extension-flexion movement at the wrist, leaning the forearm away from the body, and using a swing of the left shoulder girdle forward and backward.

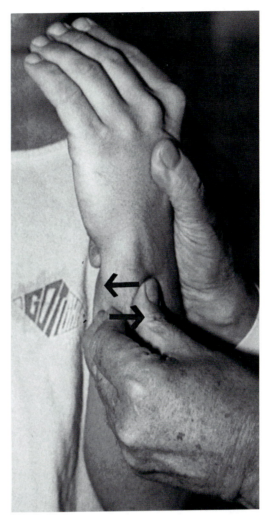

Fig. 5-71 Position adopted to elicit anteroposterior glide at the inferior radioulnar joint. The examiner stabilizes the lower end of the radius with the right hand and pushes the lower end of the ulna forward upon it with the left hand.

chapter 6

Intricacies and Interrelationships in the Body Systems

The previous five chapters are revision chapters in sequential order. Nothing contained therein counters our knowledge of anatomy, physiology, or pathology. However, I have included a few elementary facts of mechanics which are not generally reviewed in relation to the structures that allow for normal economic, efficient movement in a living subject.

This chapter is a non-sequitur to what has gone before. Its position in the book and its contents are deliberate and designed to remind the reader that nothing in the practice of medicine is really simple. There is a tendency to classify patients by their conditions. This results, sooner or later, in the patient becoming a case instead of a unique individual.

I have taken random samples of difficult conundrums in the realm of diagnosis which any practicing physician may face at any time on any day. The objective in selecting each condition is to remind the practicing physician that patients who suffer from different causes of musculoskeletal pain and dysfunction in the system do not fit neatly into some preconceived compartment. Confusing interrelationships between the body systems and the inter-twining of symptoms result in misinterpretation with leads to erroneous diagnoses.

TRIGGER POINTS

Problems of pain from synovial joints or from any part of the musculoskeletal system and from any pathologic condition that causes pain always produce some associated muscle response. This is guarding muscle spasm or splinting to prevent painful movement in the structure that is involved.

Pain that is referred to the musculoskeletal system appears to the nervous system pain centers as a symptom in the musculoskeletal system. It responds as though this were the case. Removal of the source from which the pain is referred often relieves the symptoms, which are just a somatic component of another system's illness. If this relief is delayed, morbid changes take place in the muscle. This creates circulatory problems in both the vascular system and the lymphatic system.

The pumping of muscle is essential to the efficiency of these systems.

Probably the most common morbid change in muscle that may itself become a source of symptoms of pain is the trigger point, as described by Travell.

Originally one of the characteristics of a trigger point as described by Travell was the jump sign. This was misinterpreted by almost everyone who read Travell's work to mean that the patient jumps from palpation, which reveals sensitive areas in muscle. Thus a patient who exhibited any jump during the physical examination was said to have one or more sensitive trigger points. Travell was describing a local muscle jump or twitch under the palpating examining finger. Thus the jump sign was abandoned, and muscle twitch response was substituted. The material in this chapter refers to and conforms to the original published material.

Etiology of Trigger Points

The etiologic factors giving rise to irritable trigger points are not as clear cut as those that give rise to mechanical joint dysfunction as described in Chapter 3. When one realizes that the musculoskeletal system is involved in every activity of living, this becomes less surprising.

Anything that lays abnormal stress on any muscle can activate the trigger point, whether that thing directly or indirectly assaults the muscle. The resolution of a muscle contusion may leave an irritable trigger point that becomes a primary source of residual pain. A trigger point in the pectoralis major muscle may be activated because pain from a cardiac condition sets off a reflex guarding spasm in it. Any systemic disease that customarily manifests itself by some musculoskeletal pain may activate the trigger point. Painful superficial or deep scars from accidents or surgery may also be a cause. Burns and bleeding cause irritability in a trigger point. Radicular or ligamentous pain may cause reflex painful muscle spasm, as a result of which a trigger point may become irritable. Bad work habits, chronic postural defects, and even poorly administered therapy may be to blame.

Anything that causes muscle spasm or muscle weakness, if unrelieved, causes irritability in trigger points. The presence of unrecognized diseases may maintain activity in trigger points; such conditions include subclinical collagen vascular disease, diabetes, subclinical nutritional deficiencies, and undetected foci of infection. Causes may be of psychosomatic origin, and the muscle involvement may be initiated by fatigue, stress, tension, fear, or anxiety; the list seemingly is unending, and this is a good reason why working with patients who are suffering from chronic pain from trigger points is so time consuming and requires unusual patience. When this is rewarded by relief of pain, however, it is so much better for everyone concerned than having to teach a patient adaptation to pain.

Diagnosis

The diagnosis of an irritable trigger point as a cause of pain is largely based on the recognition of a pattern of pain that the patient describes and that the examiner remembers as being typical of a trigger point in any given muscle. These patterns of pain bear no relationship to any neuroanatomic distribution. They bear no relation to patterns of radiating pain or to pain from neuritis or entrapment syndrome.

Predictability of Patterns of Pain

The recognition of the pattern of pain is the main clue to the diagnosis, and the source, being in a predictable place that on stimulation predictably reproduces the pattern of referred pain, clinches it. Then the results of treatment, if it is properly applied, are also predictable. Lasting relief from pain is achieved so long as the cause of the irritable trigger point has also been relieved. Because muscles learn bad habits quickly and unlearn them slowly, if at all, symptoms even of long standing arising from hitherto unrecognized trigger points may be relieved quite readily.

The trigger point syndrome is a clinical syndrome, and it is only recently that the so-called scientific method has led research to uncover facts to support the clinical hypothesis. Electromyography and the study of biopsy material under the electron microscope have shown predictable, even if rather nonspecific, changes in areas of muscle where trigger points clinically lie. Medical research usually eventually supports the findings of clinical research, especially when clinical findings are so predictable. Meanwhile, patients should not be denied treatment that works for lack of so-called scientific support of that work.

Figure 6-1 illustrates the common patterns of pain from those muscles that are most frequently involved in the trigger point syndrome. These are examples randomly chosen, to which readers should be able to add from their own experience as they become accustomed to recognizing trigger points. From these examples, it is easy to see how a patient's cause of pain can be misdiagnosed because the pain mimics that originating from other pathologic conditions.

The Sternocleidomastoid Muscle

Figure 6-2 illustrates the referred pain pattern from the sternocleidomastoid muscle. When the irritable trigger point is in the sternal division of this muscle, pain manifests itself in the stippled areas over the face. When the irritable focus is in the clavicular division of the muscle, the pain of which the patient complains is chiefly in the ear (indistinguishable from true ear pain) and the forehead (indistinguishable from headaches from other causes). When a trigger point is giving rise to this frontal headache, there may be a cross-reference of pain to the forehead on the other side. There may also be tooth pain (toothache) in the lower jaw, even in edentulous patients.

The Gluteus Minimus Muscle

Another muscle of particular interest is the gluteus minimus muscle. If there is an irritable trigger point in it, the pattern of referred pain is identical to the pattern of pain caused by prolapse of a fourth lumbar intervertebral disc. Often after the disc is removed this pattern of pain in the leg persists, becoming a primary source of symptoms.

Treatment by the use of either a coolant spray or local injection and stretch is bound to fail unless the physician remembers that this muscle has two functions: The anterior fibers partially function as a hip flexor, and the posterior fibers act mostly as an abductor. The stretch part of the treatment, therefore, has to be with the muscle being passively stretched in extension with adduction of the hip.

The Anterior Third of the Deltoid Muscle

There is another muscle that needs special attention. The anterior third of the deltoid muscle is different because it has three functions. It is partly a shoulder flexor, an internal rotator, and an abductor. In treating a trigger point in this muscle, the muscle must be stretched in all three directions opposite to each function (Fig. 6-3).

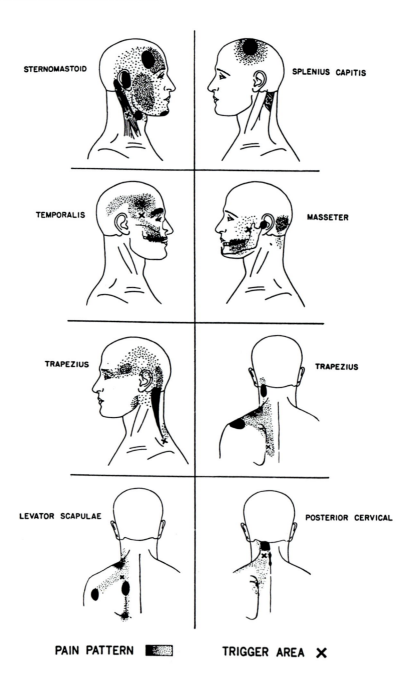

PAIN PATTERN ▮▮ **TRIGGER AREA** ✗

Fig. 6-1 Main sites of predictable trigger points in the head, neck, and posterior forequarter areas, and predictable patterns of referred pain from them. In each picture, X indicates the trigger point. The black areas indicate the most common sites of refered pain. The heavily speckled areas indicate less common sites, and the lightly speckled areas are occasional sites of referred pain. *Source:* Reprinted with permission from *Postgraduate Medicine* (1952;2:425), copyright © 1952 by Janet G. Travell.

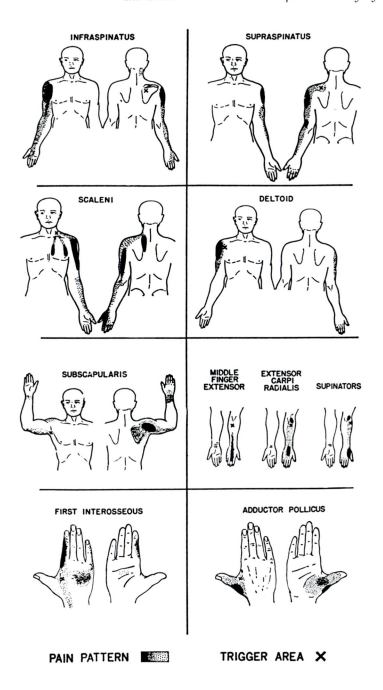

Fig. 6-1 *continued*

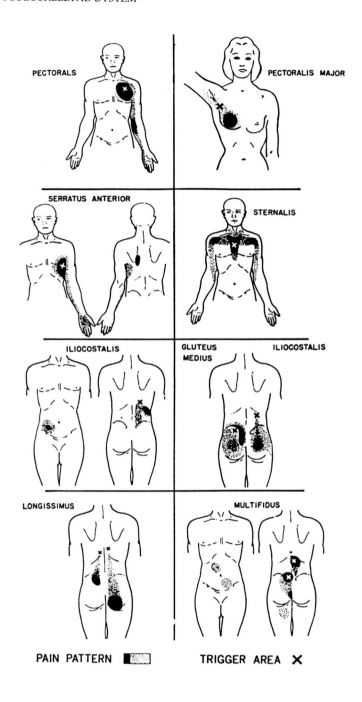

PAIN PATTERN ▓▓   TRIGGER AREA ✗

Fig. 6-1 *continued*

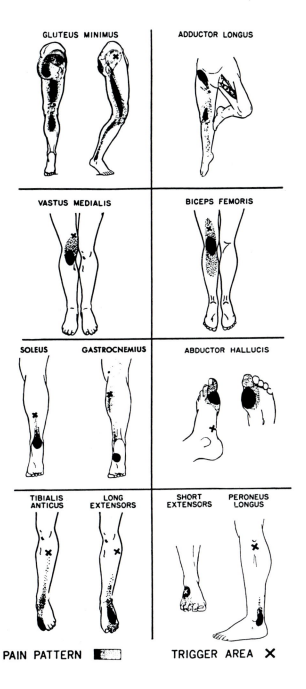

Fig. 6-1 *continued*

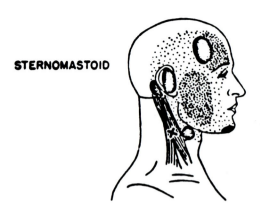

Fig. 6-2 Referred patterns of pain from trigger points in the sternocleidomastoid muscle. The sternal division refers pain chiefly to the face. The clavicular division refers pain chiefly in the ear and the forehead. There may be a cross-reference of pain to the forehead on the opposite side. *Source:* Reprinted with permission from *Headache* (1967;7:23–29), Copyright © 1967 by Janet G. Travell.

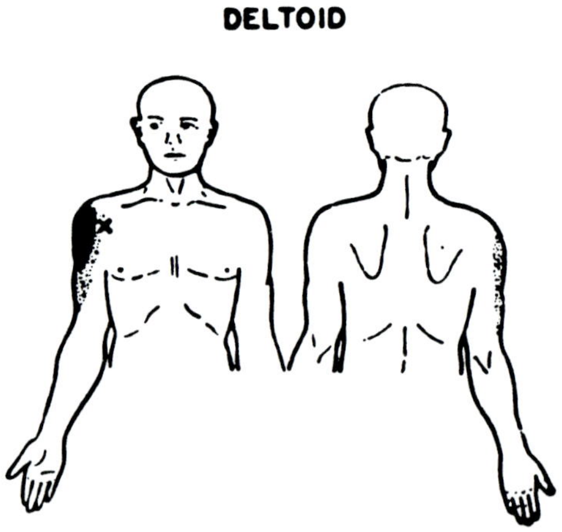

Fig. 6-3 Referred pain pattern of the anterior deltoid muscles. Because the muscle has three functions, it needs to be stretched in the three directions opposite them. *Source:* Reprinted with permission from *Headache* (1967;7:23–29), Copyright © 1967 by Janet G. Travell.

The Anterior Scalene Muscle

Special attention is drawn to the anterior scalene muscle. Because it is a muscle of the neck, one might expect the referred pain from the trigger point in it to occur in the head or the face areas. It is frequently injured, as is the sternomastoid muscle, in flexion-extension injuries in automobile accidents. The anterior scalene trigger point does not refer pain into the head and neck, however. It refers pain into the chest wall, over the shawl area of the shoulder, and down the front and back of the upper extremity laterally into the index finger and over the back in relation to the upper third of the vertebral border of the scapula (Fig. 6-4).

The pain at the vertebral border of the scapula is identical to pain arising from a prolapse of the sixth cervical disc. This mimicry might easily place a diagnostician in jeopardy. A patient with a referred pain pattern may become a chronic pain patient after the successful removal of the disc that originally appeared to cause it.

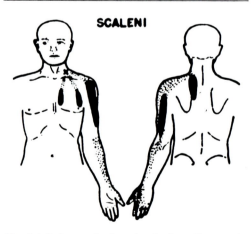

Fig. 6-4 Patterns of referred pain from the anterior scalene muscle. Note that this neck muscle does not refer pain into the head. *Source:* Reprinted with permission from *Headache* (1967;7:23–29), Copyright © 1967 by Janet G. Travell.

HEADACHES

It is surprising how seldom the musculoskeletal causes of headaches (head pains) are recognized. They are more usually blamed on stress and tension. Yet the more experience one has with trigger points, the more commonly this source of pain can be found and successfully treated.

There are 10 muscles commonly involved in the causation of headaches, 9 of which cause overlapping patterns of pain (Table 6-1). These are the sternocleidomastoid, trapezius, masseter, temporalis, splenius cervicis, cervical strap, frontalis, occipitalis, and external pterygoid muscles.

The etiologic factors giving rise to this singular condition are head pains following whiplash injuries, surgical procedures on the head and neck, dental procedures, general anesthetic procedures, visual problems, chilling of neck muscles by air conditioning or draughts, viral infections, mechanical joint problems in the upper spine, the wearing of a sling, habitual postural problems, or bad work habits. The patterns of pain from these muscles are illustrated in Figure 6-5.

Special attention should be given to the black areas in these figures, which involve the teeth, jaws, and ears. It is interesting that the pain in these locations is indistinguishable from tooth pain and earache due to local pathology. The tooth pain may occur in edentulous patients, however, and the earache may occur in people with a perfectly normal hearing apparatus. The teeth react to changes of heat and cold and on chewing.

Limitation of movement of the neck is often associated with the headaches discussed above. This may occur without coincidental joint dysfunction being present. Both these conditions may coexist, however, and joint dysfunction may be the primary cause of guarding muscle spasm with or without trigger points in the involved muscles. If both conditions are present, both must be treated.

When pain in the head arises from dysfunction of the occipitoatlantal facet joints or of the atlantoaxial facet joints, it takes on the characteristics of radiating pain from the distribution of the occipital and

Table 6-1 Muscles Producing Overlapping Pain Patterns

Type of Pain	Pain Source Muscles
Earache	Sternocleidomastoid, masseter, external pterygoid
Temporal headache	Sternocleidomastoid, temporalis, trapezius
Suboccipital headache	Trapezius, posterior cervical strap
Occipital headache	Trapezius, sternocleidomastoid, occipitalis, posterior part of temporalis
Jaw pain and toothache	Masseter, temporalis, sternocleidomastoid
Headache behind eye	Temporalis, trapezius, sternocleidomastoid, splenius cervicis
Headache above eye	Sternocleidomastoid, frontalis, temporalis, masseter

auricular nerves (which arise from the second and third cervical nerve roots) rather than the characteristics of referred pain which, when associated with trigger points is in a nonsegmental pattern.

ASSESSING PAIN AFTER NECK INJURIES

The structures of the neck are the same as those in any other part of the musculoskeletal system. The possibility of any of them being the source of symptoms after injury must be assessed. The only singular difficult problem that may make this more hazardous than elsewhere is the close relationship of neck structures with structures of other vital systems that may become involved. These are the spinal cord, the cervical nerve roots, the thalamus, the stellate ganglia, the major blood vessels to the head and upper extremities, the pharynx, the larynx, the vocal cords, the trachea, and the esophagus.

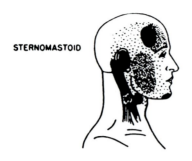

STERNOMASTOID

The patterns of referred pain from trigger points in the sternocleidomastoid muscle. The common frontal head pain (headache) may be referred to the opposite side of the head from the involved muscle.

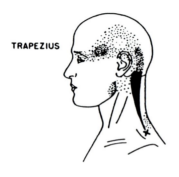

TRAPEZIUS

The pattern of referred pain from the shawl area trigger point in the trapezius muscle. Note that it is chiefly suboccipital but is frequently referred to behind the eye.

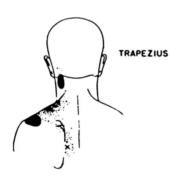

TRAPEZIUS

The pattern of referred pain from the vertebral border of the scapula trigger point in the trapezius. Suboccipital head pain may be quite intense.

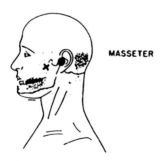

MASSETER

The pattern of referred pain from the trigger point in the masseter muscle. Loss of temporomandibular joint function is quite common when this trigger point is irritable.

Fig. 6-5

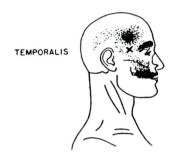

TEMPORALIS

The pattern of referred pain from a trigger point in the temporalis muscle. Toothache may be intense in the upper jaw.

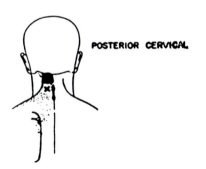

SPLENIUS CAPITIS

The pattern of referred pain from a trigger point in the splenius capitis (cervicis) muscle.

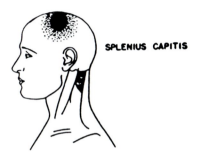

POSTERIOR CERVICAL

The pattern of referred pain from a trigger point in the posterior cervical strap muscle.

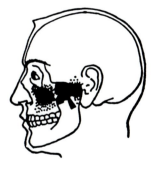

The pattern of referred pain from a trigger point in the external pterygoid muscle; sinus pain may be intense.

Fig. 6-5 *continued*

Another reason for difficulty in assessment is that most injuries to the neck are occult, showing no external evidence of trauma even when bleeding may have been severe. Internal injuries may be more threatening than obvious external signs might suggest.

Thus it is more important than ever to listen to the history carefully, to observe carefully, to palpate gently, and to move passively within the limits of pain. The pupils of the eyes should be examined, and it should be remembered that in deceleration-acceleration injuries any level in the spine, not just the cervical part of it, may be involved.

This simply reiterates the special need for the examiner to appreciate the importance of recognizing the system as it is when assessing a back problem. The examiner, by logical inference, must accept that the involvement of the system's structures in the extremities is the same as their involvement in the back, but the physical signs must be logically interpreted because they cannot be clearly demonstrated. Logic and common sense are useful clinical tools.

"Whiplash" Injury

It is the residual symptoms persisting for months and perhaps years after a patient has suffered an injury from a "whiplash" type of trauma that makes the patient feel that he or she is being carelessly cared for by those concerned with compensation. Under these circumstances the patient is usually angry and the examiner bored. This is not the way to start a good professional relationship. The subject cannot properly be judged unless it is clearly understood that there is no such pathologic condition as a whiplash injury.

It has become commonplace for the term *whiplash injury* to be used by lay people and professionals alike, and those who use it

usually exclude any symptoms other than those that arise from the cervical spine. Most often the soft tissues of the neck are excluded from their thinking, which remains limited to possible neurologic causes (eg, an injured disc, strained muscles, sprained ligaments, or a pinched nerve). One practically never hears the term *whiplash* used when in reference to injuries in any other part of the spine; it would be of benefit if it were recognized that any part of the spine may be affected in the same way when a patient is involved in any sort of moving accident, whether automobiles are involved or not. When the relief of symptoms is delayed, physicians and therapists tend to forget the original time when symptoms were first manifested and too easily fall into the habit of thinking that these symptoms persist because the patient has developed hope of considerable monetary gains. This is an unfair approach to such a patient. It is a sad commentary that physicians, lawyers, and insurance companies do not handle problems in these patients in any different a manner than they did 25 years ago.

Pursuing this line of thought, it seems incredible that those who claim to be professional scientists (or scientists in a profession) can be so unscientific as to allow themselves to continue using descriptive diagnostic terms instead of well-recognized pathologic terms that indicate changes in structures within the musculoskeletal system as the cause of symptoms.

In assessing any problem of pain arising from the musculoskeletal system, be it acute or chronic, the first determination that must be made is the anatomic structure (or structures) within the system from which the pain is arising.

The structures of the musculoskeletal system received attention in Chapter 2, where the importance of looking at the whole system is stressed. The pathologic changes that may affect these structures have been discussed, and it has been made clear that topographic fragmentation of the system in a diagnostic assessment should be discouraged.

As in any other part of the musculoskeletal system, there are two common causes of symptoms that are residual from healing and are frequently overlooked. These are simple mechanical joint dysfunction and the existence of a diagnosable irritable trigger point. One of the important differences between a mechanical pain and pain from other pathologic causes, as understood in the basic science of pathology, is that joint dysfunction describes a condition within synovial joints causing pain as characterized by loss of function without destruction of structure. In an orthodox pathologic diagnosis, loss of motion is associated with some destructive involvement of some structure.

As a result of immobilization of the neck as part of treatment of symptoms from an acute injury, the supporting muscles of the cervical spine become weak and even atrophied. Besides producing synovial joint dysfunction, this may result in irritability of trigger points in the muscles, which may give rise to bizarre symptoms of pain mimicking joint pain, headaches, and vertigo. The normal tonic reflexes of the muscles of the neck play an important part in maintenance of body equilibrium. Neck injuries may also precipitate symptoms from an otherwise innocuous cervical rib. They may also precipitate the onset of symptoms from an anomalous anterior scalene muscle.

Radiographic Findings

After injury, radiographs of the cervical spine are often reported as showing a loss of the normal lordotic curve or a flattening of the normal curve. Radiologists often say that this change is characteristic of muscle spasm. Not only is this interpretation misleading; logically, it is incorrect.

The neck is like a hunting bow. It is concave posteriorly, and the major muscles of the neck represent the bow string. If these muscles go into spasm, then the concave curve of the bow becomes exaggerated, not less curved or flattened.

The flattening of the curve of the cervical spine after an injury to the neck causes architectural changes in the spine because of painful injury to the joint. The reflex reaction of muscle to pain from joints is to go into guarding spasm in an effort to splint the painful joints to prevent them from hurting on movement. The spasm is a morbid secondary reaction that usually does not cause independent symptoms unless the primary cause of pain is overlooked and not treated. The pain may persist after the relief of the joint cause because the muscle has developed a trigger point or points that in the restoration phase of treatment may now be found to be an untreated primary cause. The interdependence of joint and muscle changes is sometimes difficult to sort out.

This radiographic change of the cervical lordosis is noted on a lateral film of the neck. Hidden in this film may be some vital information if the soft tissues, not the skeleton, are studied. There is a gray homogenous shadow in front of the white bodies of the vertebrae and the black shadow of the air passages in front. If the width of this gray shadow is more than the width of the body of the fifth cervical vertebra, the change in size is due to a hematoma if it follows trauma. In the absence of trauma, it is due either to an inflammatory lesion or to a tumor.

There is another interesting feature to note when studying the lateral film, but it requires the taking of a film with the head bent forward on the neck. The optimum safe movement in adults of the odontoid is 3 mm, and in children it is 5 mm. Anything more means laxness or tearing of the restraining ligament behind it. This may be a result of trauma or some inflammatory cause. It is particularly important to remember that no manipulative intervention in a pain-motion situation should be used if the patient has acute tonsillitis, ankylosing spondylitis, rheumatoid arthritis, or (in children) Still's disease.

There are two common and important technical errors that may be made. The first is on the open-mouth view, in which the base of the odontoid process may be obscured by overlapping bone shadows, as a result of which odontoid fractures may be missed. The second technical error is that the lateral view fails to discern the bodies of C-7 and T-1. It requires rather special techniques to demonstrate the upper three thoracic vertebrae, as a result of which an avulsion fracture of the spinous process of C-7 (shoveler's fracture) may be missed, and changes of aseptic necrosis of an upper thoracic vertebral body may also be missed. This condition may not show up for 2 or 3 years after injury; it is sometimes called Kümmell's disease.

Overgrowth of callus from a laminar fracture may intrude on the epidural space and be missed on routine films. The ligamentum flavum may hypertrophy, and both these conditions may result in spinal stenosis. Radiographs will not detect fractures in the outer facets of the joints of Luschka. There may be rotary subluxation of the axis and vertebral artery insufficiency, giving rise to the flop syndrome or other transient neurologic symptoms.

Osteoarthritis and Ligament Injuries

It is particularly important with people who have symptoms residual from neck injuries to remember that changes reported as being characteristic of osteoarthritis do not occur overnight. Most patients who are reported to have such changes radiographically have had pain-free osteoarthritis for years and will still have the same radiographic changes if they become free of pain again after a painful injury.

Occasionally, after acute symptoms of a musculoskeletal injury to the neck have subsided, a patient with symptoms that he or she considers residual from the injury has unmasked manifestations of some other disease involving the central nervous system. Such a situation poses difficult problems between physician and patient.

Ligament injuries are difficult to diagnose clinically except in the rare instances in which an interspinous ligament is ruptured and a localized interspinous step-down can be palpated. Joint or junction instability is surely caused by traumatic ligament pathology, however.

Fibrositis Scars and Adhesions

Scars from healed muscle fiber tears may give rise to pain, and after disuse myostatic contractures of the supporting muscles of the neck may also be the basis of later residual symptoms.

Fibrositis of the erector spinae muscles and the muscles attached to the scapula may be the cause of persisting symptoms. This presumably is due to the altered physiology in them by unrelieved protective spasm and atrophy. Often a distant focus of infection will keep this condition active, and treatment is ineffectual until it is found and eradicated.

Because it is not uncommon for intraarticular adhesions to occur in injuries of synovial joints of the extremities, one must postulate that a similar situation can arise after severe synovial joint trauma to the interlaminar joints of the spine. Intraarticular adhesions give rise to joint dysfunction.

Assessment of Residual Symptoms from a "Whiplash" Injury

The injury designated "whiplash" is not confined to the neck. It may affect any part of the back. If the bones, the discs, or the joints are traumatized, it is just common sense to realize that the ligaments and the muscles may also be damaged. If this is true, then it is certain that there has been intrinsic bleeding, which will not be visible from the surface of the body. Those who are accustomed to finding fault with intervertebral discs when assessing patients with spinal pain should remember that there are no intervertebral discs in relation to the first and second cervical nerves.

Just because structural changes in the extremities are easily inspected, palpated, moved, and visualized radiographically does not mean that similar injuries to the back react any differently. It means that the physician must rely more on the patient's history, symptoms, and signs elicited by clinical examination and their logical interpretation.

A common cause of residual symptoms after a "whiplash" type of injury is mechanical joint dysfunction from any area in the spine, including the sacroiliac joint. These symptoms may be well localized to a source. They may equally well be diffused and referred from the source to almost any part of the body. Another common cause is the Travell trigger point. In patients who have had symptoms for a long time, these conditions may coexist. Both of them have been discussed at length in earlier chapters. Parenthetically, it must be remembered that the costovertebral joints are part of the back and may have to be differentiated from the facet joint in the thoracic spine during the clinical assessment.

To those who are unaccustomed to thinking of the system, patients' complaints may seem to be quite bizarre and therefore unreal. As mentioned earlier, the normal tonic reflexes of the muscles of the neck play an important part in the maintenance of body equilibrium. Neck injuries may also precipitate symptoms from an otherwise innocuous cervical rib. They may also precipitate the onset of symptoms from an anamolous anterior scalene muscle.

Residual forequarter pain may, in fact, be arising in the shoulder joint of the involved side without there necessarily being any noticeable extrinsic injury to the shoulder joint itself at the time of the traumatic episode. Likewise, dysfunction in the glenohumeral joint may have occurred because of disuse (ie, movement of it caused pain in the injured neck during the acute phase of the injury, and the patient avoided its use). Radicular symptoms may be residual from a "whiplash" injury. The symptoms are just as likely to be due to capsular swelling from either synovitis or hemarthrosis in an interlaminar joint resulting from pressure as from prolapse of a nucleus pulposus.

Causalgia may be a residual symptom after a neck injury because of scarring around, or irritation of, the stellate ganglion on the affected side. Also, because of the intricate communication between the cervical sympathetic ganglia and the cranial nerves (particularly the trigeminal, the abducens, the facial, and the auditory nerves and the upper four cervical spinal nerves), patients may suffer bizarre symptoms in the head, face, eyes, ears, and arms.

COCCYX PAIN

Direct trauma to the coccyx gives rise to intractable pain that may even become worse if surgical removal of it is undertaken when all else has failed. This often produces a chronic pain situation of its own. The sacrococcygeal junction frequently shows evidence of joint dysfunction after direct trauma, and its relief by manipulative means can be almost immediate.

The normal joint play movements at this junction are those of tilting. The index finger of the examining or treating hand is placed just distal to the sacrum inside the rectum, and the thumb is placed posterially on the body surface. In this manner the first segment of the coccyx can be tilted forward and backward, and the loss of play becomes apparent. If there is associated ligament injury, immediate relief is delayed because the ligaments have to heal. Rest from function, as usual, is an essential part of treatment. This can satisfactorily be obtained by strapping the buttocks tightly together; crutches should be used for walking, and when the patient has to sit for long periods polyethylene cushions can be helpful and comfortable. If joint play needs to be restored, infiltration of the junction with procaine is recommended.

When the buttocks are properly strapped together, there is no inconvenience for the patient in toileting. When adhesive tape is used for this purpose, one should realize that it is the tension and not the adherence of the strapping that is effective. Suitable lengths of 2-inch adhesive tape are cut; they should be long enough to circle the back from one anterior-superior iliac to the other horizontally. The whole surface of the adhesive tape should be covered by gauze bandage except 2 inches at each end. A sufficient number of tapes is used so that each overlaps in the next one by a half (ie, 1 inch). Strapping starts on one side of the buttocks and proceeds to the other, so that as each tape is applied the other hand of the operator can pull the buttocks closely together while attaching the free end on the opposite side. Usually it is not necessary to maintain the strapping for more than 3 or 4 days, and where it adheres to the skin tincture of benzoin should be used to protect the skin.

THE FORWARD HEAD SYNDROME*

Postural Deviations

Changes from the normal posture of the head may result from extrinsic or intrinsic trauma, fatigue, work habits, psychologic posturing, or poorly adjusted bifocal glasses. Normally, the head's center of

---

*This section was contributed by Thomas E. Shaw, PT.

gravity is located at a point just anterior to the cervical spine and just superior to the temporomandibular joint. For every inch the center of gravity moves forward, the lower cervical spine is subject to increasing forces of compression. This is equivalent to (and therefore in addition to) the force of the weight of the head. If the head weighs 15 pounds, the head held forward 1 inch produces a compressive load in the lower cervical spine equivalent to 30 pounds of head weight. If the forward head displacement is 2 inches, then the compressive forces are equivalent to 45 pounds of head weight. The head always rules the body's position, and the body adjusts itself under the head.

If there is joint dysfunction anywhere in the musculoskeletal system that is uncorrected and affects the parallel plane of the eyes and ears and occlusion of the mandible in its horizontal plane, the head must move forward out of its normal position. These new planes are maintained at the expense of normal function almost anywhere in the musculoskeletal system. If there is a rotational or side-bending component in this aberrant posture, the head rotates away from the midline, and a compensatory scoliosis develops to rotate the head back in an attempt to restore the ability to look ahead in as near a horizontal position as possible. The cause of this abnormal posturing may be a short leg, pronation of a foot, or any uncorrected spinal anomaly.

Gravity tends to exert a force on the head and neck that makes them fall forward, even when the normal person is in the erect position. The skull balanced on the spine is a lever system with the fulcrum at the atlantooccipital joints and the center of gravity anterior to them. The counterbalance to the weight of the skull is the posterior cervical muscles. Aggravating the tendency to hold the head forward are, for instance, prolonged sitting in front of a television set, the design of office furniture (and for that matter domestic furniture and automobile and airplane seats), and even laziness.

The forward head syndrome results from these everyday hazards unless a conscious effort is made to hold the head erect. If any one of three postural planes of the head or the neck is disturbed from the horizontal positions, therapy programs must be designed to attempt to correct it. These planes are the bipupular plane (sight), the otic plane (semicircular canals and equilibrium), and the transverse occlusal plane (the position of the mandible in space). Mechanoreceptors in the mandible and the upper cervical spine react to postural changes of the mandible, the cranium, and the upper and lower cervical spines to provide sensory feedback by which an individual maintains these planes in their horizontal positions.

Functional Units

The upper quarter of the body is a functional unit made up of numerous intimately related musculoskeletal structures. To perform normally, all the synovial joints must be in their normal loose-pack position at rest when a minimal degree of compression and shear is placed on them. These joints are limited in their movement excursions by their ligaments, as all joints are, and they are moved by the muscles that act on them.

Considering the mandible (which articulates with the cranium through the temporomandibular joints) and the positional effect of it on the teeth both at rest and in function leads to consideration of what normal occlusion is. The cranium articulates with the upper cervical spine (the occiput, the atlas, the axis, and the third cervical vertebra). The cervical spine is divided into two functional units: the upper, consisting of the occiput to the third cervical vertebra; and the lower, consisting of the third through the seventh cervical vertebrae. Each segment must be considered separately to some extent. The upper cervical segment articulates with the lower cervical segment, and this in turn articulates with the upper thoracic spine.

Functionally, the upper thoracic spine acts completely or not at all, but it is convenient to consider it in segments too. The upper one, extending from the cervical thoracic spine, articulates with the manubrium sterni via the ribs. The first through third junctions are the most important functionally. The first and second ribs plus the manubrium ultimately articulate with the mandible by the infrahyoid muscle group, which attaches to the free-floating hyoid bone. The first and second ribs attach to both the upper and the lower cervical spine segments because of the anatomic position of the scalene muscles. The sternum and the clavicle attach to the occiput by the sternocleidomastoid muscles. The shoulder girdle (scapula, humerus, acromioclavicular joint, clavicle, and sternoclavicular joint) is related either through the joints to all other components of the upper quarter or through the muscular attachments to the scapula, which is attached to the occiput by the upper trapezius muscle and to the upper cervical spine via the levator scapulae. It is also attached to the lower cervical spine by the trapezius in its upper third and to the upper thoracic spine by the middle trapezius and the rhomboid muscles. There is also attachment to the ribs by the serratus anterior and pectoralis minor muscles, to the mandible by the omohyoid muscles, and to the manubrium through the acromioclavicular and sternoclavicular synovial joints. The humerus attaches to the ribs and the sternum by the pectoralis major muscle.

As stated, in the normal upright balanced position of the head on the neck, the joints are in their neutral or loose-pack position. The antagonistic muscle groups (those anterior, posterior, and lateral in the neck and upper thorax) balance the head and cervical spine without undue stress and with the least amount of energy expenditure. The shoulder girdles control the anteroposterior position of the head and cervical spine, and the scapulae are slightly retracted. The clavicles are horizontal and slightly posterior to the first rib. The lower cervical spine segment maintains a normal lordosis, and the cranium is in a slight flexion on the upper cervical spine segment. The mandible is in a neutral position with the proper resting vertical dimension; that is, the teeth are not in contact, and the condyles of the mandible are in a slight anteroinferior position within the articular fossa. The orthostatic posture resembles the old military posture: chest out, shoulders back, and stomach in.

Effects of Forward Head Position

When the upper quarter of the body falls into the forward head position, many of the component joints are taken to the extreme of a particular range of motion or put into the closed-pack position. If this position is held for an extended period of time or is frequently induced because of repetitive minor stresses, the joint capsules and ligaments are overstretched as a result of an adaptive change that occurs within and around the joints, and they ultimately lose their normal range of motion. The articular cartilage will be overcompressed, which presumably encourages its degeneration. The intervertebral discs also undergo early degeneration as a result of the increased compression and shearing forces. The antagonistic muscle groups no longer efficiently balance the head and neck. One group shortens while its antagonistic group is stretched beyond its normal resting length. All the muscles become hyperactive and prone to dysfunction and pain. Musculoskeletal dysfunctions, compressive syndromes, vascular dysfunction, and peripheral nerve entrapments may all occur, causing local or referred pain (or both) anywhere in the upper quarter.

In the forward head syndrome, the shoulder girdles (scapulae), which are the positional foundation of the head and neck, protract, elevate, and internally rotate,

causing a round shoulder appearance. The head moves forward, but to maintain the three planes of horizontal reference the cranium extends on the atlas. This causes the lower cervical spine to flex and lose its normal lordosis. To maintain the body's center of gravity, the upper thoracic spine extends, loses its normal kyphosis, and appears to flatten. This flattening makes it seem that there is an increased cervical lordosis, with extension of the cranium and upper cervical spine segment on the lower cervical spine segment. This is verifiable on radiographs.

Extension of the cranium causes the suprahyoid and infrahyoid muscles to stretch and pull the mandible and its condyles inferiorly and posteriorly, which opens the mouth. Most people subconsciously will close the mouth, inducing hyperactivity of the masseter and temporalis muscles. The mandibular condyles are then pulled posteriorly and superiorly, reducing the resting vertical dimension and putting the condyles of the temporomandibular joint into the closed-pack position. There is hyperactivity of the antagonistic muscle groups balancing the head and cervical spine, producing irritability of trigger points in the stressed muscles and dysfunction. Increased force created by the posterior cervical muscles in maintaining the head upright and keeping it from further forward movement increases compression of the lower cervical spine segment. This ultimately causes early degenerative changes in the joints and discs in the lower cervical region. The sixth cervical disc is affected most frequently and may cause impingement on the seventh cervical nerve root.

Suprascapular Nerve Entrapment

Protraction of the scapula may result in entrapment of the suprascapular nerve because it is stretched where it is tethered in relationship to the acromioclavicular joint. When the arm is elevated overhead, the nerve is further stretched, causing pain and restriction of shoulder flexion and abduction. The suprascapular nerve innervates the supraspinatus and infraspinatus muscles, and if these are weak because of nerve entrapment then suprahumeral dysfunction may develop. Good strength and endurance of the rotator cuff are necessary in glenohumeral function to maintain the head of the humerus and the larger part of the glenoid fossa when they are in function. This minimizes impingement and friction of the rotator cuff tendons and subacromial bursae between the greater tuberosity and acromial arch, which causes traumatic tendinitis and bursitis. When the scapula is protracted, it is no longer in the coronal plane but lies in the sagittal plane. What appears to be flexion of the glenohumeral joint is actually abduction, and this maximizes impingement between the greater tuberosity of the humerus and the acromial arch.

Clavicular Motion

Anterior and superior movement of the scapula causes the clavicle to move forward and slightly upward. In these patients, especially those with unilateral involvement, the clavicle is elevated and angles diagonally above its usual horizontal position. The medial end of the clavicle, as it articulates with the sternum, protrudes anteriorly. There is increased compression of the acromioclavicular and sternoclavicular joints, which may cause pain in upper extremity movement. The increased angle of the clavicle causes the first rib to tilt forward, which decreases the thoracic outlet. There are also shortening and hyperactivity of the pectoralis major and minor muscles. The pectoralis major muscle holds the scapula in a protracted position and internally rotates the humerus, which adds to the suprahumeral impingement of the greater tuberosity on the acromion because

the humerus must externally rotate when abducting to minimize friction in the suprahumeral part of the glenohumeral joint.

Occipital Nerve Entrapment

Extension of the cranium (occiput) on the upper cervical spine segment often causes mechanical compression of the posterior suboccipital structures and of the occipital nerves, which then become entrapped. This is a common cause of muscle tension headaches with facial pain. With extension of the cranium, there is an approximation of the occiput to the posterior arch of the first cervical vertebra, which approximates with the lamina and spinous process of the second cervical vertebra. The posterior rami of the first and second cervical nerves exit posteriorly and laterally, passing between these bone structures through ligaments and the suboccipital musculature. Compression of these rami by the bony and soft tissue structures or by the constant hypertonicity of the suboccipital muscles that are holding the cranium in extension will cause mechanical irritation. Patients often complain of local suboccipital pain caused by this extension, which produces the closed-pack position of the joints, particularly of the atlantooccipital joints. This may secondarily cause irritable trigger points in the suboccipital muscles. The first and second cervical nerves join to form the great occipital nerve, which innervates the top of the head. This is one explanation for headaches that shoot from the suboccipital area over the top of the head bilaterally.

Some patients complain of unilateral or bilateral supraorbital and suboccipital pain. This is because the great occipital nerve has rami communicants with the supraorbital branch of the trigeminal nerve. Some patients complain of unilateral occipital and mandibular pain because of the involvement of the second and third cervical nerve roots. Some patients may complain of unilateral pain from the occiput to the vertex of the skull; this is because the second cervical nerve root is partially entrapped, and this entrapment is aggravated by rotation of the head on the atlas and the axis. Often there are combined rotational/side-bending dysfunctions of the atlantooccipital and atlantoaxial joints, which cause functional scoliosis of the spine below as a compensation to keep the head straight, forward, and level.

Anterior Neck Muscles

Hyperactivity of the sternocleidomastoid muscles and the scalene muscles accentuates the forward head posture and causes dysfunction. When the sternocleidomastoid muscles contract bilaterally, they flex the lower cervical spine while extending the head on the atlas. In the normal orthostatic position, the sternocleidomastoid muscles lie in a plane approaching 90° to the horizontal. This may be a cause of disturbance in equilibrium.

When the scalene muscles contract bilaterally, they flex the lower cervical spine and also elevate the first and second ribs up under the clavicle. This may induce other entrapment symptoms because the brachial plexus, primarily the lower trunk, and the subclavian artery are compressed between the anterior and medial scalene muscles. The brachial plexus and artery and the subclavian vein may be compressed between the first rib and clavicle. If the lower trunk of the plexus is compressed, patients complain of pain or paresthesia (or both) in the ulnar nerve distribution in the hand. If the entire plexus or artery is compressed, the complaint is of paresthesia or coldness (or both) of the hand. If the entire plexus or artery is compressed, the complaint is of paresthesia or coldness (or both) in all five fingers. If the subclavian vein is involved, patients com-

plain of swelling or stiffness (or both) of the hand.

Both the dorsal scapula and the long thoracic nerves penetrate the medial scalene muscle; if they are compressed by constant muscle contraction, patients may complain of pain or weakness (or both) in the associated muscles. The dorsal scapular nerve supplies the rhomboids, which are often the site of pain with cervical dysfunction, but this interscapular pain may also be referred from a cervical disc or from upper thoracic interlaminar joint dysfunction. Forward head syndrome patients may also complain of axillary pain, which may arise from irritable trigger points in the serratus anterior muscle. If this produces weakness in the muscle, it also allows scapular winging to occur, which may be confused with an entrapment lesion of the long thoracic nerve.

Trigger Points

Other pain problems arise from abnormal stresses imposed by the foward head syndrome on the musculoskeletal structures. With the sternocleidomastoid muscles shortened and the levator scapulae muscles stretched as they attempt to balance the cervical spine, irritable trigger points arise in the levator muscles near their attachment to the superior pole of the vertebral border of the scapula. These cause referred pain in the shawl area of the shoulder girdle, pain behind the axilla, and pain along the vertebral border of the scapula. The attachment of the levator scapulae to the transverse processes of the atlas may cause subjection of the atlas to asymmetric rotational forces, which produce synovial joint dysfunction in the atlantooccipital joints, the atlantoaxial joints, or both. The upper cervical plexus is bordered laterally by the sternocleidomastoid muscle and medially by the levator scapulae muscle, so that its nerve roots may be irritated by mechanical friction between the muscle borders. The resulting pain may be aggravated by flexion and abduction movements of the glenohumeral joint.

The semispinalis capitis may also develop an irritable trigger point. It runs parallel to the spinous processes from the upper thoracic spine to the base of the occiput. This pain is described as hairline headaches (although the hairline may have recessed) that worsen when working with the hair, when washing it, or when combing it. Through various aponeurotic relays, tightness of these muscles may produce facial pains.

Myofascial Dysfunction Pain

Masseter and temporalis muscle dysfunctions caused by the forward head syndrome may cause symptoms of toothache, earache, tinnitus, and occlusive problems. These may cause pain because they result in shifting of the cranium from its normal orthostatic position. Myofascial dysfunction pain is a more accurate term than temporomandibular joint dysfunction because in most cases the problem arises external to the joint rather than from within it.

It should not be surprising, then, that occlusal and temporomandibular joint dysfunctions cause related upper quarter dysfunctions. When the mandible loses its resting vertical dimension and the condyles of the temporomandibular joint are in a closed-pack position regardless of where the dysfunction began, it is often necessary to give patients orthotic mandibular appliances to restore the resting vertical dimension and to balance the mandible on the cranium, which begins to balance the entire upper quarter of the body. Occlusal and temporomandibular joint dysfunctions may need physical treatment to regain the orthostatic position of the upper quarter to maintain proper occlusal and joint function.

When the cranium shifts from the orthostatic position in the anteroposterior side-bending or rotational directions, the mandible shifts and gives rise to occlusal dysfunctions. Primary occlusal dysfunctions cause the cranium to shift on the mandible to maintain the occlusal plane in the horizontal position. Hyperactivity of the temporalis and masseter muscles brings the condyles of the mandible into the closed-pack position, which leads to what is often diagnosed as atypical facial pain from the temporomandibular joint. This causes degeneration of the intraarticular meniscus which produces the clicking jaw. Degeneration of the condyles and hyaline cartilage (crepitation with movement) causes local joint pain from mechanical irritation (traumatic arthritis) and ear dysfunctions. The patient may describe noises in the ear, which may suggest a hearing loss.

Problems with Swallowing and Speech

Patients often complain of pain and difficulty with swallowing, tightness and soreness of the throat, and changes in the voice. This is because the suprahyoid and infrahyoid muscles are put on a stretch. This lessens the mobility of the larynx and upper trachea. Often the tongue loses its proper resting position (posterior to the teeth and superior against the palate), which is necessary for the proper resting vertical dimension (from the top of the head to the chin). This inhibits the action of the masseter and temporalis muscles. The proper swallowing pattern is impaired, as is diaphragmatic breathing. Patients tend to develop the infantile swallowing pattern, which adds to their oral and occlusal dysfunction. Many of these patients become mouth breathers or upper thoracic breathers, which accentuates the forward head posture because the scalene and the sternocleidomastoid muscles are accessory muscles of respiration. With the tongue against the palate, a patient is forced to breathe lazily, and this facilitates the diaphragm. This not only increases oxygen intake but also increases venous and lymphatic flow to help relieve the circulatory stasis, which may be adding to a patient's complaint of pain, and to normalize the blood pH.

Associated Spine Problems

The contracted scapulae and subsequent anterior movement of the clavicles mechanically decrease the inspirational volume of the chest and thus the oxygen intake. The patient is forced to breathe faster by using accessory respiratory muscles. This helps explain why such patients complain of fatiguing easily.

The thoracic spine responds to the forward head posture by increasing or decreasing its kyphosis, depending on how the lumbar spine and lower extremities compensate for the load. Many patients have flattening of the thoracic spine with the resultant decrease of the lumbar lordosis. These patients often have tight plantar fascia and insufficiency of lower leg ankle flexor musculature.

Other patients compensate by increasing the thoracic kyphosis and the lumbar lordosis, which leads to a dowager's hump. In any case, the head is extended on the upper cervical spine segment, the lower cervical spine segment is flexed, and the scapulae are protracted.

In treating these, the head must be rebalanced over the body. If adaptive changes have not been of long standing, improved posture can be obtained. In unilateral problems, the first thoracic junction is often rotated to the side of dysfunction. This has to be corrected because it is the foundation junction of the cervical spine. Rotation results from the contraction of the

scalene muscles on the involved side, which pulls the first ribs superiorly and posteriorly and causes the transverse process of the attached first thoracic vertebra to move posteriorly with rotation to the involved side.

Physical Therapeutic Measures

Pain symptoms arising from the forward head syndrome respond to modalities of physical therapy when they are diligently and properly applied. One cannot dramatically alter the posture of a 70-year-old patient who has had a significant forward head position for 20 years or more, but one can attempt to halt the progression of the symptoms. It is possible to alter the posture in an adolescent or young adult patient. The patient should be evaluated at rest and asleep. Abnormal posture at these times perpetuates the existing dysfunctions. A solid foam rubber pillow should not be used during sleep. The head and cervical spine must be kept in a straight and orthostatic position.

When the patient is sitting, the lumbar lordosis must be actively or passively maintained and the scapulae retracted. When standing, the patient should maintain the shoulders back and the chest up (or out). Breathing and swallowing patterns should be evaluated and treated as necessary.

Patient exercise programs should be individually tailored, but all patients should be shown the following basic exercises to restore the orthostatic position:

- diaphragmatic breathing, pressing the tongue to the roof of the mouth
- scapula retraction and depression
- nodding the head on the cervical spine only
- axial extension (keeping the head and eyes level, the lower cervical spine is pulled posteriorly in an attempt to restore the lordosis)

"Whiplash"

"Whiplash" patients often demonstrate many of these dysfunctions in the weeks after trauma because muscle hyperactivity forces them into the forward head posture. Patients without trauma but with poor posture insidiously develop individual or group dysfunctions over a long period of time. Others develop dysfunctions from a predisposition due to poor posture.

In a younger person where significant adaptive changes have not yet occurred, postural changes are possible. The clinician can successfully treat the dysfunctions discussed above, but the patient must be instructed in how to perform daily living activities and in proper posture. The patient must bear the ultimate responsibility of taking care of his or her own body and must participate actively in the treatment program.

CHEST WALL PAIN

Chest pain is a common symptom causing a patient to seek medical advice. If cardiac, pulmonary, epigastric, and breast causes are ruled out, however, few physicians pursue a diagnostic cause of this symptom, leaving an overanxious, dissatisfied patient. Musculoskeletal causes of chest pain or, more accurately, chest wall pain are numerous and, once diagnosed, are usually relieved by physical therapy.

Occult Rib Fractures

Occult fractures may occur in ribs, especially in patients with a chronic cough or in those who have had an explosive sneeze. The involved rib, being a long bone, can be auscultated to detect diminished or absent bone conduction of sound on percussion. This is diagnostic of a frac-

ture. Crepitus at the fracture site can also be palpated and auscultated.

Nevertheless, it is not sufficient to determine that there is a fracture. It must be determined whether the fracture is through a pathologic lesion in bone or through normal bone. Radiographs may be helpful. On viewing the films, the examiner should count the ribs; frequently a rib is missing from a normal-looking chest wall. In this instance, rib destruction is usually from malignant metastatic invasion. If it had been surgically removed, a scar would be noted by the examiner. This should lead to further history taking, which might uncover hidden parenchymal causes of pain. Rib pain without fracture may indicate bone tumor (such as multiple myeloma) or disease affecting bone.

Painful Scars

Scars may be painful or pain free. Keloid changes in the scar tissue may be painful. Rarely, keloid changes may be subcutaneous without being visible on the surface. There may be entrapment of sensory nerve fibrils or receptors in contracted fibrous tissue. Painful scars set off reflex guarding spasm in related muscle, which may cause pain or may set up an irritable trigger point within the muscle.

Costovertebral Joints

Acute joint dysfunction in a costovertebral joint complex after intrinsic trauma is common. It produces such acute pain that breathing hurts and walking is impaired, and the patient may be unable to sit in a chair; lying down is almost impossible. There is a method to differentiate between facet joint and rib joint complex involvement. Treatment of facet joint cannot be expected to restore play to a costovertebral joint complex.

Raney's Syndrome

Osteoarthritic changes may complicate costovertebral joint dysfunction, and the patient may not respond to any physical therapy. This complicated condition is sometimes called Raney's syndrome. The surgical removal of the transverse vertebral process and the head and neck of the offending rib may be necessary.

Shingles

A patient with intercostal radiating pain around the chest wall for which no local cause or traumatic origin is suspected may have shingles, even in the absence of skin lesions. Recent contact by an adult patient with a child with chickenpox is suggestive of this. Diabetic thoracic radiculopathy must also be considered when the lower roots are involved. The patient may present with abdominal pain as the sole symptom.

Epidural Mass

There may be more serious causes for radiating chest wall pain. It is a characteristic of an epidural mass or a spinal cord tumor. Masses in the epidural space, although uncommon in the thoracic spine, may be vascular, neurogenic, inflammatory, or caused by bleeding. The pathologic lesion is usually two levels higher than the detected sensory level. This is usually clearly defined on examination. In the back, the signs suggesting the correct level are the reaction to gentle percussion over the vertebra at the level of the lesion and intense tenderness and marked tightness on skin rolling at the same level over the spine and bilaterally over the paravertebral troughs.

A patient with an epidural abscess causing chest wall pain is obviously a sick person with high fever and other symptoms. In cases of an abscess, knowing that it is located two segments higher than the sensory level detected around the chest wall obviates the need for myelography, which is a hazardous procedure in these cases.

Border of Scapula Pain

Pain at the vertebral border of a scapula presents a complex diagnostic puzzle. It may arise from muscle; a prolapsed intervertebral disc in the cervical spine; a cervical cord tumor; adventitious bursitis; fibrositic induration of muscle from a focus of infection such as a tooth root abscess; and irritable trigger points in various muscles, particularly the levator scapulae muscle, the anterior scalene muscle, or the serratus anterior muscle. These muscle sources are discussed as they arise. The correct muscle must be identified as the source of trigger point pain for successful treatment.

Less intense pain and, less commonly, a trapezius trigger point may produce vertebral border of scapula pain also. Trigger point pain must always be differentiated from acute fibrositis. The latter may be caused by a focus of infection, and frequently local induration of muscle with pain is found in the trapezius, the rhomboids, and the supraspinatus and infraspinatus muscles.

A prolapsed disc between the sixth and seventh cervical vertebrae, or between the seventh cervical vertebra and the first thoracic vertebra, characteristically produces pain at the upper third of the vertebral border of either scapula. A cervical spinal cord tumor and, rarely, syringomyelia produce this pain.

Any respiratory viral infection may be heralded by chest wall pain, as may pleurisy or empyema. These patients must also show signs of general malaise, and the differentiation of their condition should not be difficult. Finally, vertebral border of scapula pain may arise because of an adventitious bursitis, which may occur where the scapula rubs across the angle of the fourth, fifth, and sixth ribs.

Costochondritis

The first ribs and the floating ribs are the only ones that do not have anterior synovial joints as well as posterior synovial joints. From these anterior joints, symptoms of pain may arise from pathologic causes that afflict all synovial joints. Strangely, pain in relation to the anterior joints may be referred from the posterior ones, and in these cases it is important to examine both ends of the ribs. There is a synostosis between the manubrium and the sternum superiorly, and there is a free-moving junction between the lower end of the sternum and the xiphisternum.

Medical literature overstresses the importance of a condition called Tietze's syndrome in discussions of anterior chest wall pain. The symptoms are localized to the second, third, and fourth costochondral junctions, and are associated with increased blood pressure, increased heart rate, and pain radiating down the left arm. This syndrome's symptoms are alarmingly similar to those of a heart attack except for the raised blood pressure. The source of pain in this condition is probably within the anterior synovial joints. Patients with pain related to the manubrial-sternal junction are rare, as are patients whose symptoms are related to the junction of the sternum with the xiphisternum. The causative pathology seems to be similar to that encountered in aseptic osteitis pubis.

The Pinching Rib

An unusual cause of musculoskeletal pain in the low lateral chest wall (or high lateral abdominal wall) is trauma from the twelfth rib impinging against the crest of the ilium and pinching soft tissue that lies between them. Less commonly, pain arises from impingement of the anterior ends of the floating eleventh and twelfth ribs, again pinching soft tissue that lies between them on forward bending. Use of nerve blocks with a local anesthetic often helps differentiate some of these conditions.

Occult Bleeding

Internal or interstitial bleeding is common in severe chest wall injury. Resolution of the extravasated blood must occur, and fibrosis must result. A fractured rib may perforate a lung wall, resulting in atelectasis. Fibrosis is always associated with contracture. This impairs chest wall movement, which may be characterized by painful breathing, especially on inspiration.

Interstitial Fibrosis

Retropleural fibrosis is similar to post-traumatic retroperitoneal fibrosis, but the symptoms of pain on inspiration, which the patient usually interprets as pain on exertion, become a difficult diagnostic problem. Musculoskeletal causes of chest pain on exertion are interlaminar or costovertebral joint dysfunction, frank or occult rib fractures, intercostal muscle fibrositis or trigger points, costochondritis, retropleural fibrosis, intercostal painful scars, or muscle fiber tears.

Cessation of activity, as occurs when the patient pauses to take a nitroglycerin tablet (which also relieves pain), can mislead the diagnostician, who is more likely to suspect a cardiac source of pain than a musculoskeletal one, even without electrocardiographic changes. Lung disease and pleural, pericardial, and mediastinal involvement in pathology must be differentiated from chest wall pain.

Eye Examination

An important part of the differential examination is the eye examination. The only physical sign of a superior sulcus (Pancoast) tumor may be the reverse Horner's syndrome: a dilated pupil and a widened palpebral fissure. Reverse Horner's syndrome is not singular to intrathoracic causes; it may also indicate irritation of the stellate ganglion in the neck from retropharyngeal bleeding or a tumor.

Miscellaneous Causes of Pain in the Chest Wall

Upper inner arm pain may arise from outer quadrant breast tumors, but local chest wall pain may herald any breast pathology, such as abscess mastitis or lactation problems. Posterior chest wall pain may be caused by an irritable trigger point in the posterior axillary part of the latissimus dorsi muscle.

One of the most extensive patterns of pain from irritable trigger points is the complex one from the anterior scalene muscle. This may produce ipsilateral sternal pain, anterior chest wall pain, or breast pain and vertebral border of scapula, shoulder, shawl, and arm pain radiating to the thumb and index finger. Trigger points in the paravertebral musculature and the forequarter muscles, which include the pectoral muscles and the serratus anterior muscle, also cause chest wall pain.

Flitting Pain

In late adolescence and young adulthood (17 to 30 years), flitting chest wall pains posteriorly may be an early symptom of ankylosing spondylitis. Young men are much more prone to this disease than young women, but it is not exclusive to the male. The early symptoms of ankylosing

spondylitis are often mistaken for growing pains, and flitting extremity joint pains also may be regarded as growing pains, although they may just as well be caused by rheumatic fever. The lightning pain of tabes dorsalis is one of the manifestations of neurosyphilis that is still unfamiliar to many physicians.

Flat Back Syndrome

Segmental flattening in the thoracic kyphosis with loss of intervertebral movement may also be a sign of ankylosing spondylitis, and the respiratory excursion of the chest wall is severely limited. Usually, segmental flattening in the thoracic spine is not associated with pain. It is often an early change in patients who later develop emphysema. In extreme cases, the narrowing of the anteroposterior diameter of the chest may cause cardiac embarrassment.

Increased Thoracic Kyphosis

Different age groups usually have different causes of increased thoracic spine kyphosis. In the young (16 to 21 years), the most common cause is Scheuermann's disease (osteochondrosis or apophysitis of the vertebral growth plates). This is not singular to the thoracic spine. This condition in adolescence is frequently misdiagnosed as growing pains and may even be considered part of aching and fatigue, stress, and tension.

In later life, when anterior crushing of vertebral bodies is established, the mechanisms of the intervertebral and costovertebral joints may be distorted, causing mechanical joint pain. In older patients, osteoporosis may be the pathology causing this deformity. The intensity of the associated pain does not appear to be related to the degree of deformity. Vertebrae may also be invaded by pressure from aneurysms, which cause posterior chest wall pain. Neurofibromas are a rare cause of chest wall pain. The importance of the early differentiation of these causes of pain cannot be underestimated.

Finally, diseases such as tuberculosis and infected discs, which are associated with *Salmonella* infection and heroin addiction, may also cause painful, increased thoracic lordosis.

ABDOMINAL WALL PAIN

It may be difficult to differentiate causes of abdominal wall pain from chest wall pain because of the fact that the upper middle and lower thirds of the abdomen receive their nerve supply from the tenth, eleventh, and twelfth thoracic nerves.

When palpating the abdomen, it must once more be stressed that the lighter the touch, the more one can feel. A well-trained palpator can readily feel diseased organs that are enlarged without having to resort to all sorts of tests. When patients present with acute abdominal pain, however, it is the reaction of the musculoskeletal system to the pain that the examiner has to interpret. Further, clues may be obtained, for instance, from the type of vomiting that occurs and from changes in bowel movements or habits and whether or not there has been blood or mucus in the stool. Changes in the color of the stool may be an important clue. In these cases laboratory data may be important even if they are nonspecific, but simple radiographs may be of little value. For instance, if gallstones are visible on a film, it does not necessarily mean that they are causing the patient's illness; if a kidney stone is not visible, it does not mean that it is not there.

A study analyzing 27 cases of sacral tumor revealed, incredibly enough, that it took an average of 8 months to diagnose the cause of the back pain and that no rectal examination was made on any of the subjects before 8 months had passed. The pain in each case was eventually self-limiting because all the patients died.

Pain may be referred from myofascial trigger points to the lower back and the abdomen. The patterns of pain that are set up by the iliocostalis muscles, the longissimus muscles, and the multifidi muscles are typical examples. Painful scars are not uncommon, and keloid changes in scars may occur. Joint dysfunction in any of the synovial joints from the tenth thoracic junction down to the lumbosacral junction may be the cause of referred pain. A disc prolapse may be the cause of radiating pain. There is one trigger point in the leg situated in the adductor longus that may give rise to a pattern of inguinal pain. Buttock pain may arise from the quadratus lumborum muscles, from the longissimus and the multifidi muscles, and from the iliocostalis and the gluteus medius muscles. The patterns of pain from these muscles mimic appendix pain, salpingeal pain, pain from ovarian sources, spastic colon, bursitis around the hip joint and ischium, rectal pain, sacroiliac dysfunction, kidney pain, liver pain, and even lower lobe pleurisy; this list is surely not a complete one. Recognition and treatment of abdominal wall pain has been the subject of discussion in the *Journal of the Royal Society of Medicine* (volume 83, January 1990, being the latest). That discussion by no means recognizes most of the musculoskeletal causes described here.

TEMPOROMANDIBULAR JOINT

It was sometime in 1986 that the *Wall Street Journal* published the second part of a dissertation on the temporomandibular joint, describing it as a new, fashionable diagnosis as a cause of pain. The message that the article was giving was that insurance carriers of health insurance programs were declining to recognize the condition as one of the things governed by their policies. In 1988 a local newspaper gave a large amount of coverage on two occasions to pain arising from this joint, and a television news program highlighted the condition as being something new and about which little is known.

There is nothing new about the temporomandibular joint. It is just part of the musculoskeletal system made up of the structures that were enumerated in Chapter 2. It is one of the five joints of the body in which there is an intraarticular meniscus. It would not be unreasonable to suggest that it is the most overused and abused joint in the whole body. It is subject to the same pathologic changes as any other joint, and these can be treated in the same way as one would treat any other joint once an accurate diagnosis has been made.

A popular approach to treating temporomandibular joint pain is for an orthotic to be made for the patient to alter in some way the occlusal mechanisms of the mouth. This is expected to have an indirect effect on changing the mechanisms of the temporomandibular joint from bad to better. This is similar to the common way of treating foot pain when a shoe insert support is prescribed for a painful foot. If a patient puts a foot support into a shoe in which the foot is already painful, then that pain is likely to become worse because there is no room in the shoe even for the foot. This really is common sense.

The temporomandibular joint, the foot, and everything else made up of musculoskeletal structures are in the system. Trismus is most often caused by an irritable trigger point in one or both masseter muscles, in one of the pterygoid muscles, or in the temporalis muscles. Such patients respond to trigger point treatment programs just as they do to this treatment in any other part of the system.

Joint dysfunction caused by loss of joint play is just as common in this joint as in any other synovial joint in the body. The meniscus may be displaced or injured, as it may be in the knee. Dysfunction of this joint responds to manipulative therapy just as any other joint in the system. The joint also may be the seat of the onset of some rheumatic disease. In one instance this was the first painful joint in a patient with ankylosing spondylitis. This patient had never complained of any unusual back pain, yet the radiographic changes of sacroiliitis were already present.

The reader is referred to the section on the forward head syndrome, which deals with other etiologic factors that may give rise to pain in a temporomandibular joint. This pain cannot respond to local therapy if the distant cause is not taken care of.

Because the two temporomandibular joints work synchronously all the time, it is usual to treat them together once a diagnosis is made of the structural cause of symptoms on the side of pain. This is not unique by any means in dealing with problems of the musculoskeletal system. It is a requirement for successful treatment throughout the system.

STRESS AND TENSION CONTROL

It has become commonplace for physicians to use the terms *noncompliant* or *psychologic overlay* when talking of or thinking of patients who do not respond to treatment as they would have hoped or wished. Seldom does it cross their minds that some diagnosis may have been overlooked that, if treated, might bring the relief they both were hoping for.

Psychoneurosis is a terrible label for a patient to carry; it is singular that this diagnosis is so frequently made in the absence of positive physical signs elicited by physical examination and so frequently in patients whose chief complaint arises from the musculoskeletal system.

There are four physical signs in psychoneurotic patients: a hippus reaction of the pupils of the eyes to light; sweating of the palms of the hands; exaggerated tendon reflexes in all four extremities without signs that are associated with long tract involvement in the nervous system (Hoffmann's sign in the upper extremities and Babinski's sign in the lower extremities), and a diminished pain reaction to pinching of the Achilles tendons.

Even when the physical signs support the diagnosis of psychoneurosis, this does not mean that the patient's complaints of the musculoskeletal system are neurotic. It simply means that one is faced with a neurotic patient with a problem in the musculoskeletal system who is going to require more patience and gentler handling than a normal patient. This is the same subjective barrier between physician and patient that may be present between them when the label of chronic pain patient is used for a patient who has had symptoms for a long time.

It is a clinical truism that, if a patient has developed a psychologic overlay because of chronic pain, the psychologic component is not going to respond to psychologic treatment unless the physical component of the illness is satisfactorily responsive to treatment at the same time.

In present day living stress starts early, even in the schools within the classroom, within the gymnasium, and on the field. These stresses may even be enhanced within the home. Ignoring them may aggravate the symptoms. With the stresses of everyday living for the average person caused by inflation, job insecurity, international unrest, gambling, the drug culture, gangs (the list seems to be unending), tensions are produced and are reflected in people from all walks of life. Let no one think

that the poor do not suffer as well as the rich: They probably suffer more.

These things make it the more unfair that well-to-do professionals are given judgmental powers over less well-cushioned workers to decide, usually without recourse to any appeal, whether they are sick or not.

Most studies about stress and tension control are concerned with a person's behavioral responses. A great deal is known about the visceral systems' responses, but so little seems to be known about musculoskeletal system responses. The common denominator of all these is pain, and pain in any system is associated with dysfunction of it.

So little is known about pain of, or in, the musculoskeletal system that in the past few years pain clinics have sprung up like weeds all over this country. The avowed mission of a pain clinic is to help people learn to live with pain. This aim abrogates the physician's responsibility to the patient and represents treatment by committee, not by the physician who is the personal choice of the patient. Where has the dogma of freedom of choice by a patient suddenly gone? This used to be one of the high tenets of organized medicine.

Pain clinics would be all very well were they staffed by those who are acquainted with every relievable (curable) known cause of pain in the musculoskeletal system. This is not the case, however, and this book draws attention to two common causes of musculoskeletal pain that are often overlooked in medical schools and consequently in professional offerings to patients. They are mechanical dysfunction in synovial joints and irritable trigger points in skeletal muscle.

chapter 7

Cross-Matching Structure and Pathologic Changes in Differential Diagnosis of Common Causes of Shoulder Pain

This chapter describes the mental gymnastics that should be undertaken when a physician is faced with a musculoskeletal pain in a patient who is seeking help for the first time. The glenohumeral joint is used as the example. This joint reflects almost anything that can occur almost anywhere in any patient's body, and pinpointing the source of pain in it may be one of the most intricate exercises that a physician must face in daily practice.

FRACTURES

The first thing that comes to the physician's mind when considering bone and trauma is a fracture. In dealing with fractures, too much reliance may be given to X-ray findings when the patient is first seen. Stress fractures and occult fractures may not show up on an X-ray film for 10 days to 3 weeks.

We are discussing the shoulder, and this is one of the areas in which a patient complains of pain after an injury yet in which routine X-ray examination at that time may show no evidence of a fracture being pres-

ent. The other sites where occult fractures occur, besides in the surgical neck of the humerus (shoulder pain); are the waist of the scaphoid (wrist pain); the waist of the tarsal talus (foot pain); and the head of the radius (elbow pain). Stress fractures are commonly seen at the neck of a metatarsal bone in the calcaneus (foot pain); at the lower end of the tibia or at the upper and lower ends of the fibula (knee and ankle pain). They may occur in vertebral bodies. When a vertebra is crushed, either both plates or only one plate may eventually show X-ray changes. If only the upper plate is injured, the underlying cause most often is trauma. If both plates are involved, then there is usually a pathologic condition of bone present in the vertebra.

Avulsion fractures may occur, but these usually are an indication of severe muscle injury and should be treated as such. If a greater tuberosity of the humerus is avulsed and is separated by more than 1/8 inch, however, then the best treatment for it is fixation by open surgery.

If a fracture does not show up on a radiograph, it can still be diagnosed at the time of injury in long bones by the diminution or absence of conduction of sound. For instance, to determine whether a humerus is is intact, the physician places the stethoscope over the acromion and sharply taps the olecranon of the ulna. In the presence of a fracture, the conduction of sound is diminished or absent. Clinically, an occult or stress fracture can be determined without recourse to radiographs. At the site of any fracture, there is a hematoma. Blood from this can be aspirated, and when it is placed on a white dish fat floats on the blood just as oil does on water.

The periosteum is subject to bruising in areas where bone may be unprotected by anything but skin fascia or fat. When a bruise organizes, it may produce chronic pain from recalcitrant scarring and is not easy to treat. Physical therapy modalities, if properly used, are most efficient. Suberythematous applications of ultraviolet light and histamine ionization applied through a positive disk electrode may be successful. If improperly used, either of these modalities may leave a skin burn. The periosteum may be invaded by pyogenic or granulomatous infections. In particular, tuberculosis, syphilis, and sarcoidosis should all be suspected as a cause of periostitis.

DISLOCATIONS

Even lay people can diagnose an anterior-inferior dislocation of the head of the humerus away from the glenoid. There is a large subscapular bursa to accommodate this. After reduction, the patient would have no problems if the principles of physical therapy in the healing phase were all being followed. The common methods used to reduce the dislocation are quite traumatic and may subject the capsule and the muscles (and, no doubt, the blood vessels and nerves in relation to the joint) to undue stretching and even tearing. If the manipulative examining techniques are used to relocate the head of the humerus, such trauma should be avoided.

It is the posterior dislocation of the glenohumeral joint that causes problems with diagnosis because it is not revealed by routine X-ray views, nor can the head of the humerus be palpated in any way to suggest that it has lost its proper anatomic relationship. A true lateral X-ray view of the joint through the chest provides the answer. A posterior dislocation is almost always associated with a fracture through the head of the humerus as it hooks around the posterior border of the glenoid. Closed reduction is difficult. If it is successful, the joint should be aspirated because bleeding is inevitable. Surgery may have to be invoked in the reduction process. Whichever is the case, if the patient is treated according to the tenets of good physical therapy espoused here, restoration of function should not prove too difficult. The therapist should remember that the patient has a residual synovitis and treat accordingly.

SWOLLEN JOINTS

When joints are injured, swelling differentiates them from joints that are in dysfunction. Simple trauma gives rise to synovitis. If the trauma is more severe, blood may account for swelling within the joint. These two conditions can be differentiated clinically. After the blood is aspirated, the synovium continues the production of excess synovial fluid, and this has to be treated in the same way as if there had been no bleeding.

The cause of a swollen joint may be pus, and pyarthrosis is one of the medical emergencies that may be encountered in infants and children. Once the pus is removed and the infection well controlled by antibiotic treatment, the joint may still be left with synovitis, which requires further attention before the joint can return to its normal functional state.

TENDINITIS

The most common source of pain causing shoulder disability is tendinitis of the supraspinatus muscle. This muscle is the most ill-designed muscle in the body. It has four functions to perform: It helps initiate abduction; it is an external rotator of the joint; it is the only muscle shown by electromyography to be electrically active when weight is carried with the arm by the side; and it stabilizes the joint in most of its functions when the arm is held away from the body. Its design belies its function.

In tendinitis there is a low-grade inflammatory reaction at the musculotendinous junction together with degenerative changes. The diagnosis of tendinitis is made clinically. The examiner places the index finger in a hole bounded laterally by the acromion process of the scapula, posteroinferiorly by the spine of the scapula, and anteriorly by the lateral end of the clavicle. Tenderness on palpation at this well-defined anatomic place is aggravated by initiating and at the same time resisting abduction. Because no anatomic structure has moved except the musculotendinous junction under the palpating finger, the symptom must be coming from that structure in that muscle. Tendinitis occurs in the biceps muscle in the anticubital fossa. It does not occur in the long head of the muscle at the shoulder. In this location ruptures tend to occur.

Another source of tendinitis is at the musculotendinous junction of the short head of the biceps. This is palpated in the deltopectoral groove about 1 inch below the coracoid process of the scapula. Its function is initiated by resisting the movement of the hand toward the face with the elbow bent and the forearm supinated. Flexion of the forearm at the elbow is resisted. Aggravation of the palpatory pain must be coming from the structure beneath the palpating finger—the short head of the biceps—because nothing else has moved.

Tendinitis may occur in any muscle of the body because that is the system. For instance, in the back the condition may be found at the musculotendinous junction of the sacrospinalis muscle. This pain gives rise to confusion because it is almost exactly like pain from a sacroiliac joint, a lumbosacral facet joint, a fifth lumbar disc prolapse, and a pinched nerve.

TENOSYNOVITIS OF THE LONG HEAD OF THE BICEPS

The tendon of the long head of the biceps has a sheath. It is important to differentiate whether the pain is arising from the tendon or the sheath. It has already been remarked that these two structures have different nerve supplies. Injection of the suprascapular nerve modifies or abolishes the pain if it is arising from the tendon sheath, leaving the tendon pain unchanged. The special need for accurate differentiation here is that tenosynovitis may herald the onset of disease, particularly collagen vascular disease and tuberculosis. There must be a clear history of injury before one can make the diagnosis of traumatic tenosynovitis.

TRIGGER POINTS

The second most common source of pain causing shoulder disability is a trigger point in one of the rotator cuff muscles (the supraspinatus or infraspinatus muscle).

Trigger points have been discussed at length in an earlier chapter. The differentiation between these and fibrositic nodules is important if only because trigger points respond predictably to treatment. The trigger point is usually at a site that the patient cannot localize because the symptoms do not appear at the source. The pattern of the patient's pain suggests the source from which it is referred. The physician can find it in a predictable place in a predictable muscle. Fibrositic induration or nodules have no predictable site within a muscle, nor do they refer consistent patterns of pain.

FIBROSITIS

There are 17 muscles attached to the scapula, and any of these may be infiltrated with fibrositic nodules, resulting in pain and loss of function in the glenohumeral joint. Skin rolling may localize the source, but there are no predictable patterns of pain.

Fibrositis at different times has been called different things. It is particularly confused with trigger points, and if one is treated as the other a patient gains no relief. The clinical differences have previously been discussed. The salient feature distinguishing between these two conditions is that a trigger point is always found in a predictable place in any muscle. The patient usually has no idea of the location of this source of pain. The pain pattern from an irritable trigger point is predictable. It is from this pattern that the clinician is alerted to the proper source. In contrast, the painful fibrositic nodule or a discrete area of muscle induration can occur anywhere in the muscle, and its position is quite unpredictable. There is no predictable pattern of pain referred from fibrositic induration. A properly diagnosed trigger point responds in a predictable way to a therapeutic program. The pain from fibrositis, which is usually a manifestation of a distant source of infection, only responds to treatment when that source is removed.

MUSCLE FIBER TEARS

Stressful and unaccustomed activity is a common cause of pain. The injury to the muscle may occur from repetitive small increments of some occupational function as well as from a single abnormal stress.

TEAR IN THE ROTATOR CUFF

Tendon tears and ruptures are not uncommon after injury. It is said that the diagnosis of a rotator cuff tear largely depends on the history of a fall directly on the tip of the shoulder. It is clear, however, that many people without any history of external trauma do suffer from occult tears. Because the cause is not recognized, most of these patients fall into the group of chronic pain patients.

ADHESIVE CAPSULITIS: THE FROZEN SHOULDER

All nine diagnoses mentioned, if neglected, result in a frozen shoulder. The term *adhesive capsulitis* is preferable because it indicates what is happening within the joint and provides some clue as to how the condition should be treated.

The glenohumeral joint has a great deal of superfluous capsule below the joint. This is designated anatomically as a bursa, specifically the subscapular bursa. Anatomically this excess of capsule is there to allow the arm to be raised above the head freely and without stretching it and giving rise to pain.

If any of the above conditions are neglected, this part of the capsule becomes a reservoir of stagnant synovial fluid. When synovial fluid does not circulate, it becomes sticky. In this case the walls of the reservoir adhere to each other. This, in fact, decreases the capacity of the capsule, which prevents the head of the humerus from doing all the things that it has to do automatically. The most important things are that the head of the humerus must drop downward and backward on the glenoid and must externally rotate on the glenoid. All of these are, in fact, play movements. When play is lost with concomitant loss of function, function cannot be restored until play has been restored.

All the voluntary movements of the glenohumeral joint to some degree or another are concerned with raising the arm from the side of the body to above the head. All the play movements occur in the opposite direction, mostly toward the feet. These downward movements are designed not only to restore play but also to open up the so-called subscapular bursa so that the head of the humerus can move freely within the capsule once again.

The reader should notice that none of the above nine diagnostic categories necessarily shows up on routine X-ray studies, and there is no laboratory test to confirm any of these conditions. Even pyarthrosis, which is the most urgent condition, shows no change in laboratory findings because the patients, especially children, have already been sick for a week or 10 days. They already have blood changes to indicate the inflammatory response. There is no change to reflect the complication. There is a clinical sign that strongly suggests a complication of pus in any organ system. That is the unpredicted development of sweating and a fluctuating fever. This still occurs quite frequently in spite of the advent of antibiotic therapy.

All these diagnoses, when occuring in the shoulder, are designated bursitis, but none of them is really bursitis. One cannot accept a diagnosis of bursitis in a location where there are no anatomic bursae. To diagnose primary bursitis not only requires the presence of a bursa; this structure also must be swollen, fluctuant, warm or hot to the touch, tender, and interfering with function of the joint. Primary bursitis may herald the onset of disease, of which two examples are gout and a collagen vascular disease, unless there is a clear history of trauma.

OSTEOARTHRITIS

One seldom sees radiographic changes in the glenohumeral joint that are said to be characteristic of osteoarthritis. Even the presence of such changes does not preclude examination with manipulative techniques. It has been shown previously that a patient may have painful osteoarthritis today that was pain-free osteoarthritis yesterday and, it is hoped, will become pain-free osteoarthritis once more with proper treatment.

DEPENDENCE ON THE NORMALCY OF OTHER JOINTS

There are three other joints that have to move freely before the glenohumeral joint can. These are the sternoclavicular joint, in which there is an intraarticular meniscus; the acromioclavicular joint; and the scapula, which must be free to move on the upper back. The scapular articulation with the chest wall is not a true synovial joint, but it certainly acts as one. The freedom of these joints should be assessed before the glenohumeral joint. If any of these joints are dysfunctional, they should be attended to before the glenohumeral joint.

LIGAMENT INJURY

It has been remarked that there is no useful ligament intimately connected with the glenohumeral joint. There is one nearby that, if injured, will impair movement of the joint because pain from the injured ligament is referred to the joint. The body reacts as though the joint in which the pain is felt is the structure at fault. The ligament in question is the acromioclavicular.

MENISCUS INJURY

There is no intraarticular meniscus in the glenohumeral joint, but there is one nearby that, if injured, refers pain to the joint and results in loss of function. This is the sternoclavicular joint. Usually its blockage can be overcome manipulatively.

BURSITIS

Most of what should be said about the relation of bursae to the glenohumeral joint has been said. It is interesting that there are no primary bursae in the back, which means that bursitis cannot occur in the back. Even so, adventitious bursae can occur in the back where there are kissing spines in the lumbar region and where the scapula border rides over the angles of the ribs upon which it rests. It is because of this latter problem that freedom of scapula movement on the chest wall becomes the central part of the treatment of adhesive capsulitis of the shoulder joint.

ORTHOPEDIC CONDITIONS

There is now a group of causes of pain that is more in the province of orthopedics and in which there is usually corroborative radiographic evidence to confirm the diagnoses even though the changes may take up to 3 weeks to develop. This is osteomyelitis, which may result from direct invasion or hematogenous invasion. Once osteomyelitis is established, it may metastasize to any other bone or any other organ; osteochondritis is the basic pathologic condition found in the vascular system. Metabolic disease in bone may be revealed. Neoplasms may be present and causing symptoms. The neoplasms may be primary or secondary, benign or malignant. They

may be from bone or the soft tissues. Osteochondromatosis is an example of a benign tumor of synovium.

JOINT DYSFUNCTION

Joint dysfunction may be primary or secondary, depending on the etiologic factor that caused it. Pain in the shoulder may be referred from causes in the cervical spine and neck, the chest, and the abdomen and because of systemic disease. The natural reaction to referred pain is changes in the musculoskeletal system as though the cause was in it. The diagnostician has the duty to rule out causes of pain in the musculoskeletal system and then to discover the source of the referred symptom.

The following lists are almost endless. This supports the growing belief that there should be a musculoskeletal specialty in medical education because orthopedic surgery, rheumatology, and orthopedic medicine do not cover the full spectrum of pain problems from which patients suffer.

Causes of Pain from the Neck

Shoulder pains may be referred from the neck. The following is a list of conditions in the neck with a major complaint of shoulder pain:

- joint dysfunction in a joint or joints of the cervical spine
- bone tumors and disease in a cervical vertebral body, including metastases, hemangioma, and tuberculosis
- an undiagnosed healed laminar fracture and cervical vertebral subluxation
- cervical ribs
- the anterior scalene syndrome
- spinal cord tumor

- nodes in the neck from metastases, leukemia, and Hodgkin's disease
- a retropharyngeal abscess
- irritation of the stellate ganglion from bleeding, an abcess, or a tumor
- cervical disc prolapse or neuritis and radiculitis
- fracture-dislocation in the cervical spine long after healing with residual dysfunction
- irritable trigger points in the neck muscles

Causes of Pain from the Arm

Shoulder pain may be referred from these conditions in the arm distal to the shoulder:

- carpal tunnel syndrome
- conditions about the elbow
- irritable trigger points in the upper arm muscles

Causes of Pain from the Chest

Shoulder pain may be referred from within the thorax or the thoracic spine. The following is a list of conditions in these areas that have been seen with a major complaint of shoulder pain:

- coronary artery disease
- pericarditis
- empyema and lung abscess
- aortic aneurysm
- pulmonary tuberculosis
- Pancoast's tumor (superior sulcus tumor)
- mediastinitis (nodes in the mediastinum)
- nodes in the axilla

- hiatal hernia
- breast cancer in the outer upper quadrant
- Kümmell's disease
- tuberculosis in the thoracic spine
- metastases in the thoracic vertebrae
- spinal cord tumor
- neurofibroma
- epidural abscess
- irritable trigger points in the thoracic wall musculature
- joint dysfunction in the upper thoracic spine and costovertebral joints

Causes of Pain from the Abdomen

The following conditions have been seen with a major complaint of shoulder pain:

- gallbladder disease
- peptic ulcer
- subphrenic abscess
- cancer of the pancreas
- liver disease, including an amebic abscess
- perisplenitis and ruptured spleen
- spinal metastases
- retroperitoneal sarcoma
- a dissecting aortic aneurysm

Causes of Pain from Systemic Diseases

Systemic diseases and organ changes may select a shoulder joint in which to present symptoms of pain. The following diseases may be diagnosed because of symptoms of pain initially in a shoulder:

- any disease caused by bacilli, bacteria, cocci, or spirochetes
- viral infections

- parasitic and fungal infestations
- gout
- sickle cell anemia and other bone infarcts
- Paget's disease
- multiple myeloma
- leukemia
- collagen vascular diseases
- acquired immunodeficiency syndrome
- Lyme disease

chapter 8

Management of Musculoskeletal Pain

Too often the initial reaction of both patients and physicians to musculoskeletal pain is carelessness. If the pain does not disappear, carelessness tends to change to overanxiety and fear, which are sublimated or suppressed. Thus the sufferer delays seeking professional advice. This period of indecision may be further delayed because of economic reasons and not knowing to whom to turn. This indecision may adversely affect young people for the rest of their lives. If acute problems of the musculoskeletal system were correctly treated at the onset of symptoms, there would be but a fraction of the chronic disability that one currently sees in people entering their golden years.

This is not as judgmental as it may sound because physicians are faced with a unique problem that does not occur when they are dealing with the other body systems. In our society compliance is uneconomical, and successful treatment may require a long time. If a person is stricken with acute appendicitis, there is usually no doubt that the appendix should be removed. After 10 days or so of healing, everything is usually back to normal. There is no disagreement that if the diagnosis is delayed the condition becomes life threatening. All

would agree that treatment should be undertaken.

Predictability is the key word for the diagnosis, the treatment, and the prognosis. This is not the case in problems of the musculoskeletal system because of the unpredictability of the diagnosis being made, the unavailability of proper treatment, and the inevitability of the prolonged disability in a person who apparently is not sick. Because there is so little visible evidence to corroborate what is wrong, these patients get little sympathy from anyone who has anything to do with them. Compromises are forever being demanded by family, friends, employers, and those trying to provide health care.

For these reasons, this chapter is going to be strictly limited to the discussion of the common aches and pains within the system that are not due to disease.

The essential elements of any pain management program are as follows: First, the correct diagnosis of the cause of the symptoms must be made. Second, it must be decided whether what is wrong is in the healing phase or in the restoration phase. Third, it must be decided what modality of pain control to use. Finally, to some extent the therapist must be prepared to educate the patient about the underlying pathologic process that is present. Initially some form of relaxation therapy must be undertaken, and controlled medication must be prescribed. Often nutrition must be improved, and emotional balancing may have to be undertaken.

There are those who vaunt the so-called scientific method in medicine. They accept diagnoses such as tennis elbow (for any elbow pain), bursitis (for any shoulder pain), spondylitis or spondylosis (for any neck pain), facet syndrome (for low back pain), and sinus tarsi syndrome (for any foot pain). This really is unbelievable. Reliance in any way on X-ray examinations, laboratory data, electromyography, computed tomography, magnetic resonance imaging, and radioisotope scans for diagnostic purposes in the musculoskeletal system is naive. To become believable, these investigations require expert interpretation. Yet it is acceptable that there is a built-in error factor of between 30% and 40%.

There are peculiar difficulties in studying pain problems of the musculoskeletal system that have to do with movement and support that confound the scientific method. The most obvious of them is that all movement and support functions cease with death. This vitiates the main research tools of allopathic medicine: postmortem and histologic studies.

HEALING PHASE

It has already been remarked that, when there is blood or pus in a joint, it must be removed to avoid morbid changes from taking place. These may not be possible to overcome in the restoration phase. Removal of blood or pus presents no problem when one is dealing with joints in the extremities, but there are few, if any, who can confidently aspirate a synovial joint in the back. There are physical therapy modalities that will assist in this phase of treatment.

Maintaining a physiologic state as normal as possible within a muscle or muscles not primarily involved in the diagnosed condition delays their atrophy. The atrophy of paretic muscles can be delayed for about six weeks by the use of interrupted galvanism. Muscle stimulation delays the loss of tone in the vascular tree. It also maintains the lymphatic circulation which otherwise allows puddling of lymph which becomes sticky and stagnant. This delays successful therapy in the restoration phase more than any other single cause.

PROPHYLAXIS

Prevention in medicine is surely as important as cure. The maintenance of fitness at all ages must be considered by all professionals involved in the delivery of health care.

This prevention might well start in the delivery room. As the baby is being born, few obstetricians think much about the baby's cervical spine as they pull on the baby's head and rotate it. This is especially true when forceps are used.

Pediatricians should discourage parents who show off the child's walking abilities by holding them up by their hands raised fully above their heads. It should be remembered that crucifixion death is due to asphyxiation. The gait of a normal person is swinging the arms by the side, the right arm with the left foot forward and the left arm with the right foot forward. Being walked with the arms above the head twists the child's back as the left foot goes forward with the left arm and the right foot goes forward with the right arm. This show-off habit must jeopardize any potential weakness in the developing spine.

Another example of potential iatrogenic causes of neck problems is seen in the operating room, where anesthesiologists tend to treat sleeping patients' necks with little respect, especially when they intubate them.

When patients have been on bedrest for any lengthy period and the order is written for them to get up and start walking again, not much thought is given to the flabby condition of the feet, which have been in disuse for a long time. Many patients are given paper slippers, which are difficult to keep on; thus their initial days of ambulation encourage a shuffling gait. Patients should be given their own socks and shoes, and therapists should be encouraged to tone up the feet and lower legs before unassisted ambulation is undertaken.

RELAXATION

Lip service is paid to relaxation. In fact, it is an important modality of therapy. Weightlessness allows relaxation to occur, and this can be achieved satisfactorily by hydrotherapy. In the absence of expensive equipment, bathing in a home tub is good hydrotherapy, provided that the patient has assistance and is able to get into and out of the tub.

An excellent regime to produce relaxation was devised by Jacobson. He bases his method on the time-honored physiologic fact that a minimal contraction of muscle is followed by a maximum relaxation. This method is effective in relieving both physical and mental tension. Once learned by a patient from a therapist well versed in the treatment, it can be performed independently by the patient at home.

EXERCISE

In any exercise program, the patient must be taught that warming up and cooling off are equally essential. This is just as important in training and in performance as it is in treatment and restoration. The warming up can be attained by the use of a modality of therapy that produces heat. It has been well documented that exercise in and of itself produces some acute reduction in muscle tension. Thus it is logical to assume that exercise might be a facilitating factor. It is generally understood that patients develop awareness of tension levels more easily when overall somatic tension is lower at the outset. There is a rest period, often a sleep period, after treatment that should not be disturbed.

Patients should be discouraged from doing any exercise that hurts them in any way or that they do not enjoy. In the healing phase of any musculoskeletal pain problem, it is incomprehensible that anyone can expect any active exercise program to do anything but delay healing. It is quite another story in the restoration phase of treatment. Unless patients are doing something pleasant, they will soon find a good reason to stop doing it. In conjunction with this, patients should never be asked to try to do anything beyond their capacity. This takes us back to the basic teaching of moderation in all things. A ballet dancer and a secretary can both greatly benefit from dancing, but having different capacities what is good for one could greatly harm the other.

Both in our educational system and in our sports systems, the philosophy to win at all costs leads to damaging stress and tension. In the scholastic fields, it leads to early intellectual burnouts; in sports it leads to unnecessary injuries. By ignoring moderation, we seem to have lost our unique ability of weighing the consequences of our free-will actions.

The taking of exercise must also be convenient. A patient with back pain derives little benefit if getting to treatment involves driving an hour each way to the therapy department for a half hour of treatment. It does even less good if the therapist fails to outline a regime to be followed during the rest of the patient's waking hours. Often the therapist must be concerned with the patient's sleep habits.

PSYCHOSOMATIC CONSIDERATIONS

Exhaustion, be it physical or mental, courts danger from every point of view. It threatens our ability to habilitate, and even the best-trained athletes or the most self-disciplined business persons may suddenly become uncoordinated and injured if they try to perform when they are exhausted. The ability to cope with stress is lost, and sleep may elude them.

Often the acceptance of deprivation of sleep is considered normal. Nothing could be further from the truth. Sleep deprivation only adds to exhaustion, and then anger or depression develops. When these things happen, blood pressure may go up or may swing up and down in response to normally unstressful stimuli. The blood levels of cholesterol, triglycerides, sugar, and uric acid tend to rise, and the blood tends to clot too readily. Whether this last effect is due primarily to autonomic dysfunction, resulting in arteriospasm, is moot; as far as the patient is concerned, however, it is relatively unimportant. Fluid retention is common, and resistance to infection is reduced by this. People become accident prone. Musculoskeletal symptoms abound in both the back and the extremities. Psychologic stress and tension produce musculoskeletal and visceral reactions. The reverse circuit is just as active, however.

A sense of fatigue should warn people against reaching the point of exhaustion. Physicians, trainers, and therapists should be able to differentiate the early signs of fatigue from the early signs of illness. It seems to be the case, however, that we depend on the removal of symptoms by chemical means rather than spending more time discovering their cause.

Nixon, an English cardiologist, reminds us that "bringing down the blood pressure with a drug is not the same as removing exhaustion and the smell of defeat. Inhibiting the heart's response with a beta-blocker such as propanolol is not the same as dealing with frustration, exhaustion, and despair." This is common sense, but the scientific method too often pushes common sense aside.

A further quotation from Nixon's teaching seems appropriate here:

> The more the health professionals give impersonal treatments, and select and organize themselves to have neither taste nor time for personal commitment, the greater will be the field for the counselor. In my opinion, more than half the people carrying the labels of hypertension or coronary disease could achieve healthy function if they learned how to be rid of hyper-arousal, exhaustion and sleep deprivation. A great advance would be made if they were taught nothing more than to be still sometimes, and to cultivate a healthy respect for fatigue.

Some people use medication and advocate tricks so that an injured athlete may be restored to early sport participation. This is mentioned just to be ignored. Anyone who returns too early to competitive sport ensures that sports-sickness is going to overtake him or her at an early date later in life. The decision for a patient to return to any activity should never be made solely on the basis of physiologic assessment. The Minnesota Multiphasic Personality Inventory, which was never designed for the purpose of determining the organicity of pain, is helpful in determining organicity of pain provided that the test is astutely interpreted and used in conjunction with a shrewd psychologic interview.

Nevertheless, determination of physical, medical, or surgical treatment should never rest on the results of a psychologic test. This is a clinical decision and must always rest on the shoulders of the physician or surgeon who is responsible for the diagnosis of the physical cause of pain.

MEDICATION AND PAIN

Of course there is a place for the use of medication in the management of joint pain. One cannot avoid mentioning the use of drugs in stress and tension control. If it is necessary to use narcotics in the control of pain, one must use enough of them. No pain killer, however, should ever be given to allow someone, especially an athlete, to do something he or she could not do without it. Morphine is better than Demerol. Morphine, in addition to its pain-relieving effect, produces a euphoria that has a soporific effect that Demerol lacks. Too little morphine frequently has an apomorphinelike effect, resulting in nausea and vomiting. These are highly undesirable effects for a patient in pain. It is doubtful that well-managed narcotic use ever led to addiction by itself.

It is difficult to understand how any ingested drug can be so selective as to affect muscle only. Surely all such medication must have a central effect. Relaxation can be achieved more safely by centrally acting drugs, which are more easily understood.

A large number of injectable "-caines" are available for injection therapy of musculoskeletal pain. Long-acting ones are always being sought and, when found, enjoy at least temporary popularity. It used to be taught that the "-caines" are metabolized within minutes of being injected. Thus the term *long acting* should be better defined by those who use it. Procaine (0.5%) without epinephrine is probably the best medication to use for injection therapy of this kind. Pharmacologically, in addition to its local anesthetic effect procaine has a curare-like action. This can only be of added benefit when it is used for pain relief and the consequent relief of muscle spasm.

Repeated injections of steroids into synovial joints can eventually produce Charcot's changes in them. Injection of steroids into tendons can weaken them and lead to their rupture. It has not been satisfactorily explained why steroids should be injected epidurally or intradurally for the relief of pain. Epidural injections become an office procedure if fresh 2% saline is used (it should be injected in small increments slowly, and it should be warmed). It works because of its physical osmotic effects.

There is, of course, a consensus against the use of steroids or antibiotic substances in training of humans. It makes one wonder why less good judgment is used in treatment of undiagnosed pain arising from the musculoskeletal system. Aspirin, or aspirin with codeine, is still the most satisfactory analgesic for most common aches and pains. Phenobarbital is satisfactory for short-term sedation, in spite of recent questioning of this property by the Food and Drug Administration. Elavil is a mood elevator. Taken in a sufficient single dose at night, and for short-term use, it serves well as a tranquilizer in practice.

TRANSCUTANEOUS NERVE STIMULATION

It has been suggested that transcutaneous nerve stimulation is a suitable modality to be used for the relief of acute musculoskeletal pain. Surely this is equivalent to using narcotics for the relief of acute abdominal pain before a diagnosis has been made. To mask symptoms by the use of any therapeutic modality is courting disaster for the patient. This is one of the first principles taught in therapeutics in medical school and often one of the first to be forgotten in practice.

SLEEP

It has been mentioned earlier that the therapist must be concerned with the patient's sleep habits and sleep deprivation. This may have to be attended to by the use of drugs over the short term. Again, aspirin itself may have a soporific effect on patients who are not accustomed to using it and who have vague aches and pains sufficient only to interfere with presleep relaxation. Chloral hydrate is a pretty innocuous drug, and Nembutal or Seconal is satisfactory. In some people, Nembutal has an excitation effect. This should be watched for.

SUPPORTS

In the management of joint pain in the healing phase, and keeping in mind the dogma of rest from function while healing is taking place, the use of supports must not be scorned. Splints, slings, braces, collars, crutches, and even wheelchairs must be properly prescribed. The patient must be correctly advised in their use.

In treating causes of foot pain, we should study footwear modification and the use of orthotics. Too often unsuitable shoes and the use of ill-designed orthotics cause pain rather than relieve it. A so-called foot or shoe support cannot be worn comfortably if it is placed in a shoe that already causes foot pain. Alteration of the heel heights of shoes deserves better attention than it receives. Again, looking upon pain as something different in each topographic area of the body, we must adhere to principles of diagnosis and treatment instead of fads and fashions. Our patients would fare much better.

NUTRITIONAL CONSIDERATIONS

It is surprising how little attention is paid to nutritional factors in the care of patients. A great deal of time is spent in discussing diet, but dieting and caring for nutrition are not synonymous. In one study of the effect of immobilization on various metabolic and psychologic functions of normal men, it was shown that well men can be made quite sick simply by immobilization and by lack of care for their nutrition. At the end of a 6-week period of immobilization, there was an average weight loss in each of these subjects of nearly 6 pounds of muscle protein. They suffered a loss of phosphorus, sulfur, creatine, and calcium in proportion to their loss of protein. A person requires 2 days of restoration for every day of musculoskeletal rest from function before reaching normal, if normal is obtainable.

The inferences to be drawn from this are that nutritional deficiencies in our sick and disabled should be disturbing. We are taught too little about this subject to be able to avoid these deficiencies or to know how to counteract them. The exhortation of a patient to lose weight before a surgical procedure is undertaken is usually a surgeon's "cop-out."

Too often diets are given for diseases rather than for individual patients with a disease. Nutritional considerations are for health and for patients who have a health problem.

DRUG INCOMPATIBILITY

In recent years a large amount of knowledge has been gathered and made available on the subject of drug incompatibilities and their adverse effects on blood chemistries and body electrolytes. Few appreciate the dangers of the drug management of pain. This is in fact an enormously skillful operation.

Two letters to the editor in the *Journal of the American Medical Association* on August 19, 1974 emphasize this. The first letter was authored by Robert B. Tally, MD and was entitled "Drug-Induced Illnesses." The second was from C. Joseph Stetler, whose byline stated that he was with the Pharmaceutical Manufacturers Association of Washington, DC. He discounted Dr Talley's figures on deaths caused by adverse drug reactions in 1971. He considered it ". . . more reasonable, therefore, to suggest a qualified estimate of 2000 to 3000 deaths associated with drug reactions in patients suffering from apparently non-lethal diseases." He quoted *Vital Statistics of the United States*—not available until 1972 and still the last available statistics in 1974—published by the National Center for Health Statistics of the Department of Health, Education, and Welfare, which listed 2 352 such deaths. The Commission of Professional and Hospital Activities, however, reported that the number of patients admitted ". . . with a final diagnosis explaining admission" of "adverse effects of medicinal agents" was 53,119. This would correspond to approximately 160,000 yearly hospitalizations for drug-induced illnesses, or 10 times the widely quoted estimate (quoted by Dr Talley).

Whatever the statistical truth, the inescapable fact is that the average prescriber knows little about the widespread adverse effects of medication within the consumer's body.

PAIN CLINICS

Pain clinics, which have grown up like weeds all over the country, do not answer these patients' problems properly. Most pain clinics lack some of the diagnostic knowledge that should be available to patients with musculoskeletal pain. It is the avowed object of a pain clinic to help patients adapt to pain rather than seek relief from it. Pain clinics, for the most part, represent treatment by committee. Attendance at them usually denotes abrogation of responsibility for patients' well-being by their personal physicians.

One of the high tenets of organized medicine used to be the freedom of choice of physician by a patient. Apparently the principle of having a captain of the health ship has been forsaken. Worse than that, it

seems that too often the consumers—our patients—are the object, rather than the subject, in a pain clinic. This is a sad state of affairs and really reflects an educational gap that has yet to be filled. This is another reason why therapists must be encouraged in structural diagnosis before initiating treatment of patients.

Some years ago a woman wrote to the *Miami Herald*, asking what she could do about her 42-year-old husband's worsening back pain of more than a year's duration. The "Ask The Doctor" column recommended trying a pain clinic. The author's description of such a clinic, which "specializes in conditions that have proven to be unresponsive to traditional medical care," failed to suggest that the diagnosis should first be reviewed. The columnist wrote:

> The Center's program emphasizes treatment in a therapeutic community that encourages participation in everyday activities and non-isolation. For instance, meals are only served in the dining room, patients are not "permitted" to stay in bed. They have to make their own beds, clean their own rooms, and do their own laundry. Help may only be sought from other patients. Activities are scheduled for 16 hours a day. The program starts with four weeks on an in-patient basis on an average, and then progresses to an out-patient program geared to the needs of the individual which "permits a transitional period between residential treatment and the resumption of independent living."

If the program fails, there is no suggestion that the patient's diagnosis should be reviewed. It is really illogical to suppose that a clinic can achieve in about a month what physicians, chiropractors, hypnosis, and drugs have failed to help in more than a year. A patient who is treated along the lines described above is to be pitied. Undoubtedly, this patient was sick.

chapter 9

Consideration of Physical Therapy Modalities

Because so little is taught in most medical schools about the modalities of physical therapy, one cannot pretend to fill this educational gap in a work that by no means purports to be a technical therapeutic treatise. This knowledge is already available in physical therapy textbooks.

The usual prescriptions for modalities that are to be used on a patient are given to a therapist by a physician. They are usually limited to ultrasound, heat, maybe cold, and some form of routine exercise program. A word should be said about the proper use of these modalities.

GENERAL PRINCIPLES

If a modality of physical therapy is prescribed for any reason other than for the reasons of its properties—namely to effect rest from function in the structure in which the pathologic condition is situated, to maintain as normal a physiologic state as possible in the structures only secondarily affected by the primary pathologic condition, to prevent morbidity, and (when healing has occurred) safely to restore any lost function—then physical therapy is being abused.

ULTRASOUND

Ultrasound is a source of deep heat; all energy is eventually converted by the body into heat. The advantage of the deep heat produced by ultrasound is that it is not concentrated by metal implants, as it is when diathermy is used. Indeed, patients with disc prolapses and nerve root involvement are often made worse when diathermy or ultrasound is used over the troubled area. Deep heating is contraindicated when patients have osteoporosis.

Another property of ultrasound is that the permeability of semipermeable membranes is increased, so that it is useful in dispersing collections of fluid within the system. This is especially true in the inaccessible synovial joints in the spine and in cases where occult bleeding has left residuals.

Ultrasound has the effect of micromassage and may be used to soften scar tissue that may be causing pain. Under water it may lessen the symptoms from plantar warts and from Dupuytren's contracture in the hands and the feet. It may be used selectively over stubborn fibrositic nodules in muscle.

Ultrasound is able to introduce drugs locally through the skin for their anti-inflammatory or analgesic properties. This therapeutic use of ultrasound is called phonophoresis. If ultrasound is used for any reason other than one of these four, it is being misused.

EXERCISE

Recent advertisements on television are saying that most physicians assess back pain by how far a patient can bend down. If this is the case, then the question must be asked as to why they prescribe routines of flexion treatment. Routine prescriptions for undiagnosed pain are usually unsuccessful. To give a patient a pamphlet illustrating the prescribed exercises being done by a young, healthy, and attractive model can scarcely be useful to a middle-aged, out-of-shape, weekend "do-it-yourselfer" who suddenly develops acute pain somewhere in the musculoskeletal system and frequently in the low back.

Therapeutic exercises may be assisted, unassisted, or resisted. They may be concentric accelerating, or shortening decelerating exercises. They may be done prone, supine, sitting, or standing. They may be for the purpose of strengthening or for the purpose of restoring useful function (a good functional result may be an imperfect anatomic but pain-free result).

No exercise should be prescribed for a patient by those who are unable to perform the prescribed exercises themselves. No therapeutic exercise, especially in the healing phase, should be performed if it is painful to the patient or if the patient appears to be clinically worse after the treatment than before. This is especially true if the worsening occurs during the night or on the following morning. In the healing phase, exercises prescribed must be tailored to fit an individual patient.

When training back muscles, however, it is almost impossible to teach them to do the same thing. This need may be fulfilled by the use of alternating current (electrical

stimulation) together with ultrasound by means of the Medcosonolator. This comes as close to the passive maintenance of a normal physiologic state as is possible in muscle, in the vascular tree, and in the lymphatic system.

To a much lesser but nonetheless important extent, interrupted galvanism does the same thing for paretic muscles, but only for about 6 weeks. Electrotherapy and muscle training are professional skills that should not be relegated to an assistant or an aide.

Lack of attention to the muscles in the healing phase also delays the loss of tone in the vascular tree. Exercise maintains the lymphatic circulation; otherwise there is puddling of lymph, which becomes sticky and stagnant. Impaired lymphatic circulation in the healing phase delays successful therapy in the restoration phase more than any other single thing except excessive fibrosis.

During the restorative phase, exercises may be done in classes, but only after supervising therapists have themselves examined each patient for undiagnosed causes of pain and for the individual's suitability for class work.

The performance of any exercise with metronomic rhythm defeats its purpose. It contradicts the physiologic cycle of muscle action, which requires the completion of the relaxation and refractory periods before a contraction period is usefully undertaken.

Patients will only follow through with an exercise program if they feel that it is doing them good. Any exercise program must be convenient and enjoyable if it is to be continued.

SYNOVIAL JOINT MANIPULATION

Earlier in this book it was stated that the primary forms of treatment used for patients suffering from musculoskeletal pain arising from a structure within the system should be a well-designed program of physical therapy. In the section on joint dysfunction, it was stated that manipulation designed to restore normal joint play, when its loss is the primary cause of symptoms, is the treatment of choice. No other therapeutic approach has any hope of predictably relieving such a patients' symptoms.

If the joint dysfunction is of long standing, there are morbid changes in other structures of the system. These must be attended to, sometimes before the manipulation, sometimes after it, and sometimes coincidentally with it. The course of treatment is determined by the therapist. Except when joint dysfunction is the primary cause of symptoms, there is no place for manipulative therapy during the healing phase. Conversely, there is scarcely a patient who would not benefit from manipulation in the restorative phase at some time or another.

SPRAY AND STRETCH FOR TRIGGER POINTS

Treatment with the coolant spray and passive manual stretching of the affected muscle may be the only treatment required to restore normal resting length. A home physical therapy program involving gentle heat and gentle eccentric lengthening-decelerating exercises continues the therapeutic process.

ELECTROTHERAPY

Iontophoresis with copper as the active ion and the current adjusted so that the anode is the active electrode cures athlete's foot. The heavy metals are fungicidal. Zinc promotes the production of granulation tissue. Procaine may be used under the anode, as may histamine and mecholyl. Hyaluronidase, being an enzyme, does not ionize. It has the property of attaching itself to the positive ion of a salt and thus can be introduced into a local area when the anode is the active electrode. In addition, when the anode is the active electrode, the current has a pain-relieving effect. Iontophoresis with the cathode as the active electrode is used for the introduction of the halogens through the skin. They have the property of softening scar tissue.

Anodal galvanism used many times a day on paralyzed muscle delays its atrophy for up to 6 weeks. Subtonal faradism relieves chronic pain of bone disease. This is the basis of the therapeutic use of transcutaneous electrical nerve stimulation. The apparatus for this modality was at one time given out indiscriminantly to patients with any kind of recalcitrant musculoskeletal pain, and its use is now severely restricted by edict of third-party payors. This modality of treatment is still useful in patients with some of the chronic pain symptoms arising from neurologic causes.

MASSAGE

Massage is probably the most time-honored modality of physical therapy, yet in the late 20th century it is probably the most denigrated of the modalities in the United States. This is because it has been abused in so-called massage parlors and because of spurious claims that it may substitute for exercise and assist in weight reduction. These are poor reasons for abandoning its professional uses.

Three types of massage are taught: effleurage, pétrissage, and tapotement (colloquially this is called hamming and damming or clapping). There is no place for tapotement in the treatment of musuloskeletal conditions arising from injury or disease. Its chief usefulness is in toning up normal muscles and, under special circumstances, in some pulmonary diseases to help clear congested lungs.

Pétrissage

The classic description of pétrissage is that the skin is picked up between the fingers and subjected to intermittent pressure. Skin rolling, cupping massage, and any form of kneading or stretching massage are included under this heading.

Skin rolling has been described earlier as a diagnostic test, especially in assessing patents with back pain; if tightness and tenderness are diffuse, then it becomes a form of therapeutic massage as part of a well-designed physical therapy program. If the envelope of the system is too tight and painful, it interferes with the function of the systems that it encloses. If manual skin rolling produces too much discomfort, initially cupping massage may be substituted for it.

Skin rolling is performed over the back by picking up the skin and superficial fascia between the thumbs and fingers and pulling the skin backward over the advancing thumbs as they move up the back, maintaining the pressure of the roll all the time. For some reason, this is not effective when the rolling crosses the back or when it is directed from the head downward.

When suction massage has to be substituted for skin rolling, a breast pump is used over a liberal application of petroleum jelly on the skin to maintain the suction. The cup is rhythmically moved over the skin up and down over the painful area. The suction can be adjusted to the tolerance of the patient.

Friction Massage

Friction massage is not a comfortable modality of treatment, but it is effective when muscle, interstitial tissue, and fascia are involved in the program of treatment for tight, painful scars. Because it is an irritable form of treatment, its use should be followed by effleurage after each session to promote relaxation.

Sustained pressure over a sensitive area of muscle appears to block noxious impulses, thus producing reflex relaxation and relief of pain. This alone is unlikely to produce any lasting change but may become part of a well-designed physical therapeutic program.

Effleurage

Effleurage is stroking massage that may be lightly or heavily performed. The light form is used to produce physical and psychologic relaxation. It also has an effect on the vascular system, improving the blood flow through injured areas. Some patients, and especially those in older age groups, may find effleurage irritating, in which case its use should be abandoned. Some people find this sort of treatment addictive; for this reason it is unwise to promote its use among the patient's family members, especially the spouse.

Heavy stroking massage is used for its mechanical effect on the vascular and lymphatic systems.

Edema Massage

Stasis in the lymphatic system because of disuse presents a major problem in the restorative phase of physical treatment, especially when there has been no instruction of patients in the healing phase to maintain as much as possible the effects of draining of a dependent part. For instance, when there is swelling in a lower leg after immobilization, edema massage must be given with an antigravity assist by positioning the patient properly. The deep massage must then start at the upper end of the involved limb and progress down to its distal end. The strokes of therapeutic massage are always performed in a centripetal manner.

TRACTION

When traction is in order for treatment of orthopedic conditions in the extremities, the physician has a choice between skin traction and skeletal traction. Traction is not used as an examining procedure in the extremities. Examining for joint play movement must not be confused with traction. Traction is exclusively a therapeutic maneuver. The lumbar and cervical spine presents the physician with a choice of skeletal traction, skin traction, or traction by the use of halters. The focus here is on the use of traction as a physical therapy modality.

In this context, therapeutic traction is best produced manually so that the therapist can monitor the reaction of the patient's tissue to pulling. Traction cannot be achieved against a curve. When it is used for some problem in the cervical or lumbar spines, their curves must first be flattened. In the cervical spine, this entails moving the chin to the neck (this does not mean lowering the chin). To flatten the lumbar spine, the knees and hips are flexed.

To achieve therapeutic traction on the cervical spine, the neck is supported by the pulling hand. The hypothenar eminence lies beneath the nuchal line of the skull, and the thumb and index finger rest on each shawl. The other hand guides the chin, neither lifting nor pulling. The traction is achieved by the examiner with the body and not the arms, first taking up the slack and then gently pulling (no jerking). This movement produces long axis extension of the joints at junctions from the occiput down to the first thoracic vertebra.

It is common sense that capsules, ligaments, and muscles cannot be stretched beyond the point of normal movement of the joints regardless of the poundage of the pull. The rules of performing joint play movement must be followed. The height of any person cannot be increased by more than the height of one and one half bodies of a cervical vertebra. This means that there is less than ⅛ inch of movement at each junction.

Traction with head halters becomes intolerable to a patient after about 20 minutes. If the therapist's hands are too small for the patient's head, a convenient and comfortable way of achieving traction is by using a carefully folded Turkish towel.

HEAT

For all practical purposes, physicians are used to using either superficial heat or deep heat largely because of the convenience of the source most readily available and not because of any special properties of either. The main thing is to recognize the properties of heat and also to realize that its therapeutic effect is not dependent on the time period of its application. There are indications for the use of heat, and there are contraindications for its use, just as there are in any other therapeutic modalities used in medicine.

Circulatory and Metabolic Properties

After an initial short vasoconstriction, vasodilation and hyperemia rapidly occur. This results in an improved blood supply to and from the part being treated. If too much heat is given, congestion occurs, which is a morbid state. If the application of heat beyond this is used, then the heat may actually produce tissue changes that result in "cooking" or frank burning.

The metabolism of the heated parts is increased. If the catabolites are not removed because, for instance, of impaired circulation or neglect, morbidity results. Heat promotes sweating, which is one way to improve the excretion of waste products resulting from disease or increased metabolism. Heat increases the threshold of sensory nerve endings. When the source of the pain is a neuritis, however, the pain may be aggravated. If a feature of the patient's condition is loss of sensation, then burns can occur in the area being treated. Warmth is relaxing to most patients, and psychic relaxation may occur. This helps promote physical relaxation.

Special Uses of Heat

Since the advent of antibiotics, most young physicians have come to believe that this is the beginning and end of all infectious diseases. It should be useful to remember that diathermy promotes healing in a way that cannot be due only to its local deep heating property. Drainage of pus still takes precedence over any other therapeutic modality. In osteomyelitis, when drainage has been achieved diathermy promotes healing. In cases of gonococcal arthritis, prostatic or pelvic diathermy promotes cure of the disease and relief of pain. In cases of sinusitis, diathermy promotes healing. Reflex heating is of value in the overall management of vascular disease because direct heating may severely complicate the disease. Diathermy is effective in treating non-specific muscular chest wall pain, and it hastens the resolution of unresolved pneumonia and abscesses in the lungs.

Most hot packs are too heavy. If a patient has to have heat applied and the applicator is too heavy, then the muscles in the area being treated work to support the weight rather than relaxing, which is the intent of the treatment.

COLD

The therapeutic uses of cold are to stop bleeding and to reduce the morbidity that may otherwise follow an acute injury. Cold also relieves pain and the muscle spasm that may be associated with it. It may also temporarily relieve spasticity, and, of course, it induces hypothermia. The physiologic effects of cold are vasoconstriction, local anesthesia, the production of a histaminelike response within the skin, and contact irritation.

Spray and Stretch Technique

Cold is applied by the use of coolant sprays, but these work best when the spray is a jet stream. The only safe spray is a mixture of fluoromethanes, which is available as Fluori-Methane (dubbed inert by the Food and Drug Administration when properly used). The fluoromethane mixture is not flammable or explosive, nor does it have anesthetic properties. The Gebauer Company puts it up in 4-ounce bottles that have a fine calibrated nozzle that emits a jet stream. It should be looked upon as ice in a bottle. It is not absorbed through the skin; its action results from the impact of the jet stream and the sensation of cold on the skin, which compete with noxious impulses from muscle spasm or trigger points.

If the muscle being treated is chilled, its spasm becomes worse. If the muscle being treated is overstretched, the pain becomes worse. The object of the treatment is to separate the muscle from its message center so that it relaxes; then it can be passively stretched to its normal resting length, which is a pain-free state. Usually, this spray and stretch treatment is part of a well planned physical therapy program, but occasionally one application is sufficient to obtain relief from symptoms.

Ice Massage

Ice massage is especially effective in the treatment of tendinitis. To apply this, an ice cube is held in a face cloth (not the usual container). The melting of the ice safeguards that the area being treated does not get too cold. The face cloth is used to mop up the cold water from the melted ice, which otherwise causes shivering. The corner of the ice cube is used, and the stroking may be back and forth over the involved musculotendinous junction.

The patient's response to ice massage is predictable. There is an initial response to cold, but this is followed by a feeling of burning, aching, and finally numbness. As soon as the skin is cold there is a histaminelike reaction, which is intensely red; this is contrary to the blanching that one expects. As the treatment continues the skin area may become corrugated, and at the site of pain a pea-sized tender mass can be felt under the ice. The strange thing is that this mass is not palpable by the examining finger. This phenomenon disappears after four or five treatments, at which time the patient's pain appears to be permanently relieved.

A prerequisite to a successful treatment is that the muscle that is primarily involved must be restricted to its pain-free limit of motion during its healing phase.

HYDROTHERAPY

Hydrotherapy has the following properties. First, it is a cleansing therapy; second, it has the property of producing weightlessness; and third, it provides gentle heat and massage.

The weightlessness produced by water allows assistive exercises to be done by patients, and it allows for relaxation. The relaxation is used in the healing phase as well as at the beginning of the restoration phase of treatment as a prelude to instituting walking or other sensible all-body activity.

There is one account of a physician who treated a series of patients who had had surgery for fractured hips. Within a day or

so of the surgical procedure, they were put in a tank of warm water up to their necks and allowed to take steps in the walking tank. The healing time of the fractures was cut down to 6 weeks, and the postoperative complications were, to all intents and purposes, eliminated.

The presence of salts in the water is of little significance. Salt water, because of its specific gravity, is more bouyant than tap water. At spas the water may contain sulfur, which promotes superficial circulation and sweating but may be an irritant to the skin. The warmth of the water promotes relaxation. Too much time in too-hot water may cause older patients to collapse. If the water is agitated, it acts as a massage. Because of its relaxing properties, it is also a pain-reducing muscle treatment when muscle spasm is a prominent feature of the patient's condition.

Whirlpool baths are a two-edged therapeutic sword after surgery or in treating an injured extremity after trauma. If the extremity is placed vertically in the whirlpool, the heat and massage properties may increase congestion and swelling.

Contrast baths are a time-honored therapeutic modality used to stimulate the vascular tree and are invaluable in treating pain arising from muscle that has a deficient blood supply from disuse. They may be contraindicated if the lack of blood supply is due to arterial disease. The part to be treated should be immersed in hot water for about twice the length of time that it spends in cold water. Each treatment should not last more than 15 minutes, and the final immersion should be in the cold water.

ULTRAVIOLET LIGHT

Ultraviolet light is bactericidal, which may be an important adjunct to the healing process in the healing phase. In the restorative phase, however, it has several important actions that are frequently overlooked.

Body ultraviolet light therapy without tanning should be used for its tonic effect in proper utilization of vitamin D in the ergosterol cycle, and it should be considered an important adjunct in the treatment of patients with senile osteoporosis, whatever drug or hormonal therapy is used. Ultraviolet light may be used as a counterirritant in the treatment of painful deep scars that follow periosteal bruising. This is especially common at the elbow and the ankle.

INJECTION THERAPY

Local anesthetics are used diagnostically and therapeutically. Steroids are almost routinely added to them. This is a fashion rather than a need. Overuse of steroids in joints leads to Charcot's type of joint destruction. Steroids in tendons may result in weakness and rupture. Steroids irritate trigger points. There are more containdications to the use of steroids than there are indications. Their use should be for some well-identified therapeutic purpose.

Injections of local anesthetics are used in conjunction with some physical therapy modalities. Largely they are used for their anesthetic effects, although procaine itself is said to have a local curarelike effect on muscle at the site of injection. Local anesthetics injected into painful ligaments are effective in relieving pain to allow stress radiographs to be taken to rule out ruptures.

Local anesthesia is used for nerve blocks to differentiate the source of pain by knocking out the sensation of one structure and leaving another unchanged. An example of this is the differentiation between pain in the biceps tendon at the shoulder and pain in its capsular tendon sheath. Infiltration on the suprascapular nerve eliminates pain from the capsule but not from the tendon.

When Sudeck's bone atrophy is the cause of pain, as it frequently is in cases of reflex muscular dystrophy, autonomic infiltration interrupts this type of pain, allowing the inauguration of a physical therapy program. Infiltration of the stellate ganglion is used when the bone atrophy is in the hand. A posterior tibial nerve block is used when the bone atrophy is in the foot. A lumbar sympathetic ganglion block is used when there is some vascular deficit in the leg. The use of procaine without epinephrine in the treatment of trigger points is discussed in Chapter 6.

After aspiration of blood or pus from a joint, its replacement by air is a pain-relieving modality. While the needle remains in the joint, the syringe is removed from it. Air is sucked into it through several gauze dressings, which may or may not act as a filter. The syringe is replaced by the needle, and the air is injected. In the past, acid potassium phosphate with procaine and lactocaine (lactic acid with procaine) were used satisfactorily for the same purpose.

When injection of fluids is used for treatment of pain arising from the musculoskeletal system, the smallest amount of fluid is used that is compatible within the area of pain. Too much fluid distends soft tissue, which in itself is pain producing, and when a trigger point is being treated by injection too much fluid just irritates it further.

Epidural injection of 2% saline into the epidural space, both as a diagnostic and as a therapeutic tool, is an innocuous, safe, and logical procedure that relies on the science of physics. The 2% solution is freshly prepared and sterilized and is warmed before use. The injection is made through the sacrococcygeal hiatus. Up to 60 mL of injection fluid is used unless the reproduction or aggravation of pain symptoms precludes this. The fluid is injected slowly and in small increments.

Before the injection is started, the straight-leg raising test on the painful side is performed with the patient supine. The patient then turns face down with two (or more) pillows under the pelvis to make the sacrum as horizontal as possible. After the skin is thoroughly cleansed, a skin bleb is raised with 1% local anesthetic through a 26-gauge needle. A needle tract is infiltrated down to the hiatus.

The saline injection is made with a 2-inch 22-gauge needle attached to a 20-mL syringe and is inserted at an angle of about 45° to the skin. A small additional amount of local anesthetic may be used until the needle is felt to have satisfactorily entered the epidural space. At that time an aspiration is undertaken to be sure that the venous plexus has not been entered. The dural sac may rarely extend this far; it would be detected by aspiration of spinal fluid. One should temporarily abandon the procedure if blood is aspirated and abandon it entirely if spinal fluid is aspirated.

If the needle is not in the epidural space, the skin over the sacrum starts to balloon almost as soon as the saline injection is initiated, and the needle should be repositioned.

There are two predictable results of the injection. The first makes it a diagnostic test. Fluid is incompressible, so that, if there is something in the epidural space that should not be there (disc material or a tumor), when the injection fluid meets it it is compressed, and the symptoms of which the patient complains are reproduced or made worse (particularly radiating leg pain).

The second result is that the sciatic symptoms may be relieved. This is probably due to the osmotic effect of the hypertonic saline withdrawing edema fluid from the involved nerve root. The straight-leg raising test is immediately repeated, and the sign may be completely negative. It may only show partial improvement, however. In this case, subsequent injections should produce relief. It is rare that one has to perform more than three injections on a patient to obtain relief of pain if the first injection produced partial relief without aggravation of the pain at the time of injection.

In postsurgical patients, relief is probably obtained by the release of epidural adhesions around a nerve root, again because the fluid injected, being incompressible, tears them.

If one believes that a bulging disc is a cause of a clinical syndrome, then one could accept the possibility that the incompressible fluid pushes back the bulge. This would be a third reason for therapeutic success.

ASSISTIVE DEVICES

There are some assistive devices that are useful adjuncts in the treatment of musculoskeletal pain on a temporary basis. As such, they can be considered a modality of physical therapy.

Crutches

The use of crutches merits more attention than is usually given to patients. Physicians tend to assume that anyone knows how to use crutches and that any crutch can be fitted to anyone. In fact, crutches can become a handicap instead of an assistive device. Axillary crutches should not be used under the axillae either for ambulation or for something to rest upon. They should be fitted to each individual so that the handpiece maintains the elbow at a 30° angle. The hands are weight bearing, not the axillae. Patients should be warned that rubber tips act as skates on wet, smooth surfaces. Loftstrand (Canadian) crutches are more useful to younger people. They allow for more activity of the arms while they are being used. If there is to be no weight bearing on one leg, however, it is easier to lose one's balance with these crutches than when using underarm crutches.

If the patient needs crutches, then it is better to use two than one. This maintains the balance and often prevents falling. Patients almost always need to be taught how to use crutches. Their use depends upon the various reasons for which they are prescribed. Many patients consider the use of crutches a label of disability. The therapist should try to educate such patients away from this concept.

Walkers

There are people who cannot be trained in the use of crutches. For them the walker is the best assistive device for ambulation. These cannot be used by older people who have to get around without weight bearing on one leg. Walkers should be high enough to keep the patient upright.

Wheelchairs

If safe relief from weight bearing cannot be attained with one or the other of the above devices, a wheelchair should be provided. For temporary use, no expensive gimmicks need be added to a model that has adequate footrests and swivel wheels at least 6 inches in diameter in front. It must have efficient brakes. Pneumatic tires are not required. People using a wheelchair for the first time require education.

Braces

Braces are too expensive to be prescribed for temporary use. Plastic braces, if available, are useful in problems of muscle weakness below the knee, however.

Splints

The judicious use of splints may be a necessary adjunct to therapy in the healing phase. When they are prescribed as a tem-

porary measure, patients must be advised about the necessity of maintaining as normal a physiologic state as possible in every structure of the musculoskeletal system except the one that is involved in the primary pathologic condition. Patients should be educated to know that immobilization produces as much mobility as functional use during the healing phase. Passive movement within the pain-free range is almost always helpful.

Collars and Spinal Braces

Collars and braces, if used correctly, are a benefit to patients as short-term devices. They should be considered adjunctive to other modalities in a well-planned treatment program. They may be soft or hard. Neither one really supports anything but rather acts as protective consciences.

For some patients with recent acute low back pain, a flexion plaster jacket may be an invaluable first-aid appliance to be worn for 3 to 5 days. When it is removed, the patient is easier to examine, which leads to the correct diagnosis of the cause of pain. Proper diagnosis opens the way for a predictable prognosis.

Figure 9-1 shows a useful method of strapping for a painful low back as a first-aid modality.

In a similar way, a Turkish towel can be wrapped around the neck in lieu of a collar. This is much more comfortable for the patient if something has to be used at night. The towel can be held together with a large diaper pin. Anything more sophisticated has little place in everyday practice.

A leather or webbing belt 2 inches in width with a three-prong buckle can be a useful assistive device. It is worn over the shirt tails with its upper border underneath the anterior-superior iliac spine. The belt should be horizontal to the floor. This constrains the sacroiliac joints and the lumbosacral junction, providing relief of low back pain as a first-aid measure.

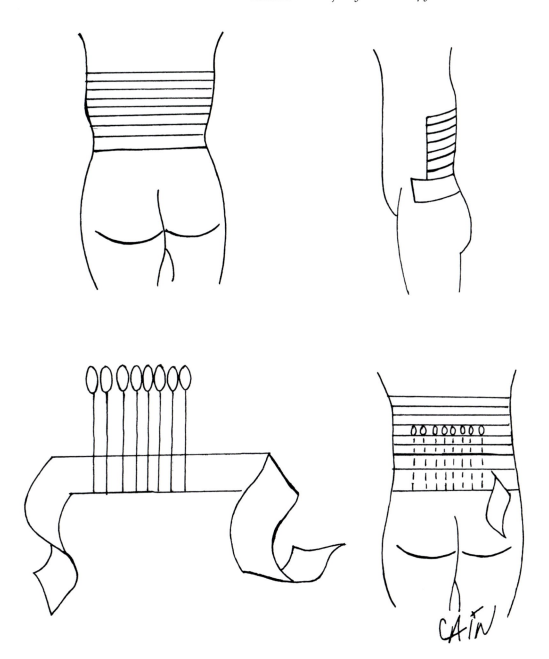

Fig. 9-1 Strapping the low back. The lowest strap has its upper edge just below the anterior-superior iliac spines, much like a pelvic band. Successive strips of tape are started from alternate sides of the body, and the tape from the other side is pulled across the midline gently but firmly.

chapter 10

Conclusion

Perhaps in this book I have gone to unusual lengths to give credit where credit is due. I feel that the nature of the book, and the nature of the works being credited warrant this treatment. To my readers I can say with certainty that the musculoskeletal system is a fact, and this unequivocal statement is based on 50 years of study. Joint play is the basic scientific feature of the system that makes it indestructible. It is a hierarchic system that must be appreciated and studied to alleviate suffering caused by its dysfunctions.

His Royal Highness the Prince of Wales gave a speech to the British Medical Association on the occasion of its 150th anniversary which included the following quotation:

> I often have thought that one of the less attractive traits of various professional bodies and institutions is the deeply ingrained suspicion and outright hostility that can exist toward anything unorthodox or unconventional. I suppose it is inevitable that something that is different should arouse strong feelings on the part of the majority whose conventional wisdom is being challenged, or, in a more social sense, whose way of life

and customs are being insulted by something rather alien.

> I suppose, too, that human nature is such that we frequently are prevented from seeing that what is taken for today's unorthodoxy probably will be tomorrow's convention. Perhaps we just have to accept it as God's will that the unorthodox individual is doomed to years of frustration, ridicule and failure in order to act out his role in the scheme of things, until his day arrives and mankind is ready to receive his message: a message that he probably finds hard to explain, but that he knows comes from a far deeper source than conscious thought.

Now rarely does a month go by without an authoritative article being published on how beneficial manipulation may be for low back pain. This does nothing to help our consumer. Until causes of pain are diagnosable, predictability of treatment remains a lottery. The manipulative lesion must be accepted.

The principles underlying the use of manipulative examination and treatment techniques bear reiterating. Any musculoskeletal examination is incomplete unless an assessment is made as to whether the play movements in the synovial joints are normal or impaired. Patients cannot perform play movements by the use of their voluntary muscles.

Patient symptoms most often are topographic. Most physical signs arise from one structure in a multi-structure system. Individual examination techniques must eventually get down to the individual play movements in one joint, on one side, and one movement of the joint at a time (occasionally in this latter instance this is not possible for technical reasons). In the back, the physical signs should be limited to one intervertebral junction or one sacroiliac joint. Gross external trauma may affect more than one level, but this should become clear from the patient's history.

An example of this is found in studying the wrist. If the play movements of the radiocarpal joint are imparied, the patient's symptoms are the function of flexion at the wrist, and a painful wrist. If the midcarpal joint is at fault, then the patient's symptom is the loss or impairment of function of extension.

If both of these functions are lost, the cause is most unlikely to be mechanical. This sort of thing is true throughout the musculoskeletal system. Simple loss of play which produces the mechanical diagnostic joint dysfunction seldom if ever impairs all voluntary movements of that topographic area. If more than one movement in that topographic area is impaired or lost, it is most unlikely that the cause of symptoms is mechanical.

Remember that all joint play and movements are less than ⅛ inch in any plane in any joint. It should be clear that no force need ever be used when restoring any play movement which has been lost. Gentleness is success; force is injurious. Remember that the lighter you touch the more you can feel.

The Validation of the Diagnosis "Joint Dysfunction" in the Synovial Joints of the Cervical Spine

INTRODUCTION

Innumerable patients seek advice because of pain in their arms, in and around their shoulder joints, in their neck and in their heads. They receive descriptive diagnoses which have little or no bearing on pathological changes that are allegedly unsupported by physical signs. For these complaints they are prescribed either analgesics, nonsteroidal anti-inflammatory drugs, or tranquilizers, possibly with some nebulous form of physical therapy usually designated "conservative treatment."

If any of these patients are unfortunate enough to have any pain in the chest they are often diagnosed as having some mild cardiac abnormality especially when they give a history of precordial pain on exertion.

Surely the time has come when we should recognize that there is nothing mysterious about the back—it is just another part of the musculoskeletal system. The structures in the back are essentially the same as the structures in the extremities. When structures of similar kind, wherever they are in the system, are affected by the same pathological changes, the same history, symptoms and physical signs, one would expect to see similar diagnoses. We are complacent with patients who come to us complaining of symptoms in the extremities; we should be able to do at least as well when they come to us complaining of symptoms in the back. Even if we cannot directly handle the structures of the back, logic and common sense should allow us to interpret similar history, symptoms and signs when they occur in the back, and arrive at the same diagnostic conclusion.

Confounding patients with diagnoses which bear no relation to demonstrable pathological change should be discouraged. When we treat patients without knowing the pathological cause underlying the patients complaints, it should not be surprising that the results of treatment are so often unpredictable.

The intent of this paper is to draw attention to the diagnosis of a mechanical cause of pain from synovial joints, known as joint dysfunction. Joint dysfunction presupposes the presence of mechanical play,

Source: Reprinted with permission from *Journal of Manipulative and Physiological Therapeutics* (1990;13[1]:7–12), Copyright © 1990, JMPT.

which is a prerequisite for normal efficient motion in anything that moves including the human body. When we talk of "play" in human synovial joints we call it synovial joint play. When joint play is lost, joint function becomes impaired and painful (1).

There are three constant etiological factors associated with this mechanical pathological condition: a) intrinsic trauma; b) immobilization, with which disuse and aging must be considered; and, c) factors residual from the healing of some more serious pathological condition. It should not be surprising, therefore, to seek a mechanical treatment to restore normal play by mechanical means when mechanical dysfunction is the primary cause of symptoms. This mechanical treatment is joint manipulation. Treatment is solely designed to restore play movements. Because they are not under the control of the voluntary muscle system they can only be restored by a second party. The prerequisite of successful treatment is, of course, learning what is normal in every synovial joint in the body. Patients cannot predictably restore lost play themselves by any form of exercise therapy or other self-imposed regimen.

To help to validate this hypothesis, manipulative examining techniques have to be used in addition to the physical diagnostic procedures that are usually taught. This unanimity of examining techniques in a multi-center study is vital if the participants are to obtain predictable clinical pictures. Only then can the result of treatment be predicted and the effectiveness of the treatment be assessed. It is impossible to examine the normal function of joints after death or to study the normal function of living joints by using the tools currently available. But does this differ from the usual research requirements which are the basis of analysis of the effectiveness of any surgical procedure? It is illogical to suggest that research on the function of the mus-

culoskeletal system can be studied by double blind methods.

METHODS AND MATERIALS

This paper is based on the study of 100 consecutive cases of "neck" patients culled at one time when I was in private practice.

Though it was unusual for these patients to complain of one symptom only, it was possible to determine a predominant symptom by which they were divided into clear cut groups for the purpose of analysis. There were seven patients who were exceptions to this, but there was no reason to drop them from the study.

Method of Examination

This report is not intended to be a handbook of examining manipulative techniques. The examination techniques used on every one of the patients in this report are explained in a previously published text (2).

The symptoms designated are: a) pain in the neck, b) pain in one or both arms, c) pain in one or both shoulder girdles, d) pain in the head or headaches, e) the fifth group is made up of the seven patients who lacked a sufficiently predominant symptom to include them in one of the other four groups.

These 100 cases are analyzed on the basis of: a) sex incidence, b) age incidence, c) duration of symptoms, d) the part played by injury at the onset of symptoms, e) an analysis of radiological reports as given by radiologists, f) a discussion of the cases in which disc degeneration was stressed in the radiological reports, and g) an assessment of the results of manipulative treatment.

RESULTS

Just over two-thirds of the patients were women (*Table 1*). One might speculate that there may be some connection between this fact and a theory that the wearing of high heels by women increases their cervical lordosis which predisposes to interlaminar joint strain and dysfunction, which I have postulated many times.

Over 50% of the patients were in the middle age group, i.e., between the ages of 40 and 60, which might be expected. Comment on the question of age and the suitability for manipulative treatment will be made later (*Table 2*).

The analysis of the time during which these patients had been suffering from their symptoms appears to be of little sig-

nificance in itself. However, reference should be made to the commentary later in this paper in which it is noted that there is no evidence that the duration of symptoms affects the expected prognosis resulting from elective manipulative therapy (*Table 3*).

Table 1 Sex incidence

	Male	Female	Total
Pain in neck	16	34	50
Pain in one or both arms	3	10	13
Pain in one or both shoulders	3	4	7
Pain in head (headaches)	9	14	23
Mixed symptoms	1	6	7
Totals	32	68	100

Table 2 Age incidence

	Age in years							
	10–19	20–29	30–39	40–49	50–59	60–69	70–79	Total
Pain in neck	3	4	5	12	15	7	4	50
Pain in arm(s)			1	7	4	1		13
Pain in shoulder(s)		1	2	2	1	1	1	7
Pain in head		6	4	8	4	1		23
Mixed symptoms			2	3	2			7
Total	3	11	14	32	26*	10	5	100

*One patient suffered from dual involvement.

Table 3 Duration of symptoms

	Days	Weeks		Months		Years						
	0–7	1–4	1–3	3–6	6–12	1–2	3–5	6–10	11–20	21–40	41	Total
Pain in neck	5	2	4	6	7	8	6	4	4	3	1	50
Pain in arm(s)			2	2	4	1	1	1	1	1	1	13
Pain in shoulder(s)			2		1		2	1			1	7
Pain in head		1		1			2	5	8	4	2	23
Mixed symptoms		1		1			1	4				7
Totals	5	4	8	10	12	9	12	15	13	8	5	100

Table 4 Relationship of symptoms to prior injury

	History of concussion	History of head injury	History of severe neck injury	History of general injury	No definite history of injury	Wry neck	Totals
Pain in neck	5	4	5	7	27	7	50
Pain in arm(s)	1		1	1	10	1	13
Pain in shoulder(s)				2	5		7
Pain in head	4	5	2	4	12		23
Mixed symptoms				1	6		7
Totals	10	9	8	15	60	8	100*

*Several patients reported dual involvement.

Table 5 Analysis of radiological reports

	Osteoarthritis	Disc degeneration	Fracture-dislocation	No abnormality detected	Other disease	Lost lordosis	Not X-rayed	Totals
Pain in neck	3	16	4	14	2	2	9	50
Pain in arm(s)		3		7			3	13
Pain in shoulder(s)	1	1		1		1	3	7
Pain in head	2	2	2	5	4	4	4	23
Mixed symptoms	1	2		1			3	7
Totals	7	24	6	28	6	7	22	100

The part played by injury in the production of symptoms is analyzed. It is remarkable how few of the patients recalled any injury which might have precipitated their symptoms. Less than two-thirds of those whose predominant symptom was head pain (headaches) remembered having any head injury or concussion. This lack of recall of injury in 50 patients supports the belief that intrinsic rather than extrinsic factors more commonly cause symptoms in the cervical spine (*Table 4*).

Only the predominant X-ray changes reported by the radiologist are noted in this analysis. For instance, in a case in which disc degeneration was reported, osteoarthritic changes were also frequently reported. In such a case the predominant feature is considered to be the disc degeneration, and the patient is recorded in this category. No attempt is made to note how often polyspondylitis marginalis osteophytica was reported as osteoarthritis, but my experience is that this is commonly done, and is often diagnostically very misleading.

Of the six patients under the heading "other disease," one of the patients in group 1 had Still's Disease, and the other had osteoporosis. Of the four patients in group 4, two patients had spina bifida occulta, one had osteoporosis and one had changes which were reported to be due to rickets in early life (*Table 5*).

Joint dysfunction, the diagnosis for which manipulative treatment is the treatment of choice, cannot be determined radiologically. It can be inferred in the cervical spine when there is a segmental loss of the normal cervical lordosis in the absence of other gross radiographic, change which are characteristic of bone or joint disease.

Method of Therapeutic Techniques

The diversity of radiological diagnoses in this group of 100 patients, whose symptoms for the most part responded to manipulative therapy (*Table 6*), emphasizes the importance of careful clinical examination and evaluation which is stressed throughout the text.

In 24 of the patients, 49 discs were reported to show marked degeneration. This does not include the patients who are categorized as having fracture-dislocations in whom, of course, there are two disc lesions each; one above and one below each fractured vertebra. On the basis of these radiological reports, these patients had been told that little if anything could be done for them. Clinical examination, however, revealed that the patient's signs were elicited at levels other than those at which the disc degeneration was reported. The results of manipulative treatment directed at the levels from which signs were elicited, rather than at levels of disc degeneration, supports the hypothesis that disc degeneration alone rarely has any bearing on a patient's symptoms. To make a diagnosis relying on the radiological appearance alone, whether CT scan, MRI or myelography may be very misleading. At the time of this study, I had not seen more than 15 cases in which a prolapsed cervical disc was the cause of symptoms (3). In each case the diagnosis was clinically clear, and surgical removal of the disc produced a cure. None of these cases occurred in this series.

DISCUSSION

Of the 100 patients under review, only 83 were subjected to manipulative treatment to relieve their symptoms. The symptoms were determined clinically to be arising from joint dysfunction in one or more of the

Table 6 Levels of disc degeneration reported in 24 cases

Between 2nd and 3rd cervical vertebrae	1
Between 3rd and 4th cervical vertebrae	4
Between 4th and 5th cervical vertebrae	7
Between 5th and 6th cervical vertebrae	19
Between 6th and 7th cervical vertebrae	14
Between 7th cervical and 1st thoracic vertebrae	4
Total in 24 cases	49

synovial interlaminar joints in the cervical spine. Thirteen patients refused manipulation and in four cases there was no indication for this form of treatment. Anesthesia (sodium pentothal) was used at the time of the initial therapeutic manipulation in 32 patients. The only reason for the use of anesthesia is to obtain muscular relaxation, which allows perfect control of the manipulative movements being used.

Neurological symptoms were present in 21 patients. However, in only three of these were there any neurological signs. In each of these three patients it was possible to make a diagnosis of neurological disease. One patient had syringomyelia, but the pain in his neck was due to joint dysfunction and not to his disease. This emphasizes the fact that a patient's symptoms are not necessarily part of a pre-existing disease. This is especially true for those patients in whom imbalance from neurological causes so easily produces joint strain and resulting joint dysfunction, which gives rise to symptoms.

The average follow-up in the patient who underwent manipulative therapy is 2 years. This is a short period but it is sufficient in a clinical appraisal of effects of treatment in patients who previously have complained of unremitting pain for a considerable length of time. In this series, 73 of the patients had symptoms for longer than 6 months, 61 of them had symptoms for longer than a year, and 52 of them (more than half the group) had symptoms for 3 years or longer.

Table 7 Results of manipulative treatment

	Cured	Marked improvement	Moderate improvement	No change	Manipulation not advised	Manipulation refused	Totals
Pain in neck	15	13	7	2	4	9	50
Pain in arm(s)	5	3	3	1		1	13
Pain in shoulder(s)		4	3				7
Pain in head	5	6	7	2		3	23
Mixed symptoms		3	4				7
Totals	25	29	24	5	4	13	100

After considering Table 7, which analyzes the clinical results of manipulative therapy, it is apparent that age is no contraindication to this form of treatment. The oldest patient treated in this series was a man of 73 years of age. Nor does the length of time for which the patient has suffered symptoms seem to have much bearing on the prognosis. However, it would be foolhardy to expect a patient who has had symptoms for 20 years to respond as dramatically as one who has only suffered for 20 days. The most dramatic cure in this series was a lady who had suffered severe and progressive symptoms of head pains, tinnitus and vertigo for 41 years.

Table 7 analyzes as objectively as possible the clinical state of the patients who were manipulated at the time at which the analysis was made. While only 83 of the 100 patients are thus reviewed, license is taken reporting these figures in percentages. Twenty-five patients, or 30% of those treated, claim to be cured of their symptoms. Of these 25 patients, the eight cases of "wry neck" were completely relieved of their symptoms immediately. In the remaining 17 cases "cured" denotes complete freedom from symptoms, but does not mean that they did not have recurrences of their symptoms following subsequent unguarded strains to their necks. However, any such recurrent attacks were also completely relieved as they occurred. Each of these 17 patients was among those who had suffered from their symptoms for

prolonged periods before I initially saw them. Each recurrence was heralded by a precipitating traumatic episode.

Twenty-nine patients, or 34% of those treated, claimed to be markedly improved. In these cases relapses were not infrequent, but the recurrent symptoms of pain were relieved without difficulty. Each relapse was precipitated by a fresh traumatic episode. Twenty-four patients, or 29% of those treated, claimed to be moderately improved; their symptoms were less aggravating than before treatment.

The Use of Anesthesia in Manipulative Therapy

In the course of my career I have manipulated hundreds of patients under anesthesia. I would choose nitrous oxide or pentothal. The former is sufficient for patients with joint dysfunction in the joints of the extremities; the latter is better when the joint dysfunction is in some joint of the spine or in one of the sacroiliac joints. I use it to obtain pure relaxation, for pain relief and sometimes for expedience—never so that I may use more force or any different technique. When using anesthesia it is not necessary to use an operating suite nor is it necessary to use any additional drug which might interfere with respiration (4).

I have never understood why my colleagues frown on this practice when they can see nothing wrong when a dentist uses these aids in their offices to facilitate difficult dental work or for the removal of teeth.

My manipulative techniques are exactly the same with the patient awake or asleep. It is interesting that when asleep the patient's restricted joint movement (amount of loss of function) is exactly the same as when he/she is awake.

So long as the therapeutic techniques are directed only at restoring joint play movements which are less than ⅛ of an inch in any one plane within the capsule, and only one joint at a time, and only one movement at a time is performed, no harm can come to any patient providing the diagnosis is clear. The manipulator must remember that no functional movement is forced and no topographical area is treated. It should also be remembered that fingers, glenohumeral joints, hip joints and knee joints should only be fractionally manipulated: i.e., a little at a time. Lost joint play movements are confined to within the synovial joint capsule.

CONCLUSION

When a patient is anesthetized, the therapeutic techniques used are exactly the same, though they are performed even more gently. They are quite specific for every synovial joint in the body. The exact therapeutic techniques have also been previously described (2).

A study of 100 patients who had symptoms arising from their cervical spines is presented. Ninety-six of these patients were deemed to have interlaminar joint dysfunction after thorough clinical examination following the criteria I have previously described (5). Eighty-three of the patients were subjected to manipulative treatment to relieve them of their symptoms.

The duration of these patients' symptoms ranged from 1 day to 41 years. Seventeen of the patients had suffered for less than 6 months and all of these were cured of their symptoms. Thirty-seven of the remainder were markedly improved and entirely satisfied with the results of their treatment. Twenty-four patients, though only admitting moderate improvement, claimed that they received more relief from manipulative treatments than any other treatment to which they had been subjected. Evidence is presented to show that the age of the patient and the duration of their symptoms has little bearing on the results of manipulative treatment.

The 44 patients who had their symptoms for longer than a year had all been treated by almost every other modality of physical therapy including traction and immobilization procedures other than fusion, without satisfying relief. Manipulation brought them this relief. This paper not only helps document the mechanical diagnostic entity of joint dysfunction but also validates the logic, common sense, and usefulness of manipulative therapy; no exotic and expensive ancillary tests (myelograms, CT scan, or MRIs) could be of any use in arriving at the correct clinical diagnoses of the clinical condition causing the patients' symptoms.

REFERENCES

1. Mennell JB. *The science and art of joint manipulation*. Vol 1. London: J & A Churchill Limited, 1945.

2. Mennell JM. *Joint pain*. Boston: Little, Brown and Co., 1964.

3. Mennell JM. Assessment of residual symptoms from a whiplash injury. In: *Proceedings of the Fourth International Congress of Physical Medicine*. 1965;107:528–29.

4. Mennell JM. Manipulation therapy for low back pain. In: *Advances in pain research and therapy*. Vol 3. John J. Bonica et al., eds. New York: Raven Press, 1979.

5. Mennell JM. *Back pain*. Boston: Little, Brown and Co., 1960.

Bibliography

Burrows HJ, Coltart WD. *Treatment by Manipulation*. Eyre & Spottiswood for the Practitioner, 1939.

Cyriax J. *Textbook of Orthopaedic Medicine*. Baltimore: Williams & Wilkins; 1969.

Ghormley R. *Collected Papers*. Mayo Clinic. 1933;25:813.

Goldthwaite JE. *Body Mechanics*. Philadelphia, Pa: JB Lippencott; 1934.

Grieve G, ed. *Modern Manual Therapy of the Vertebral Column*. London: Churchill Livingstone; 1984.

Hammer W, ed. *Functional Soft Tissue Examination and Treatment by Manual Methods*. Gaithersburg, Md: Aspen Publishers, Inc.; 1990.

Jacobson E. *Progressive Relaxation*. Chicago, Ill: University of Chicago Press; 1974.

Jostes FA. Place of manipulative procedures in the overall treatment rationale for painful back conditions. *Arch Phys Med*. 1944;25:716–720.

Magnuson P. *Ring the Night Bell*. Boston, Mass: Little, Brown and Company; 1959.

Marlin T. *Manipulative Treatment*. London: Edward Arnold & Co.; 1934.

Melzak R. Prolonged relief of pain by brief, intense transcutaneous somatic stimulation. *Pain*. 1975;1:357–373.

Melzak R, Wall PD. Pain mechanics: New theory. *Science*. 1965;150:971–979.

Mennell JB. *Backache*. London: J & A Churchill; 1917.

Mennell JB. *Physical Treatment by Movement, Manipulation, and Massage*. 3rd ed. London: J & A Churchill; 1934.

Mennell JB. *The Science and Art of Joint Manipulation: The Extremities*. 2nd ed. London: J & A Churchill, 1952.

Mennell JB. *The Science and Art of Joint Manipulation: The Spinal Column*. 2nd. ed. London: J & A Churchill, 1952.

Mennell JB. *Treatment of Fractures by Mobilization and Massage*. New York, NY: Macmillan; 1910.

Mennel JM. Backache. *N Z Med J*. 1947; 46:324–331.

Mennel JM. *Back Pain—Diagnosis and Treatment Using Manipulative Techniques*. Boston, Mass: Little, Brown and Company; 1960.

Mennell JM. Clinical evaluation of low back pain and its treatment. *Arch Phys Med Rehabil*. 1955.

Mennell JM. Common problems of foot pain. *Patient Care Journal*. March 15, 1975.

Mennell JM. Diagnosis and treatment of myofascial pain arising from trigger points. Paper presented at the 1st AAATC International Interdisciplinary Conference on Stress and Tension Control.

Mennell JM. Epidural injections in the treatment of sciatic pain. *Orthop Rev.* 1975; Comment and Reponse.

Mennell JM. *Foot Pain.* Boston, Mass: Little, Brown & Company; 1969.

Mennell JM. History of the development of medical manipulative concepts. In *The Research Status of Spinal Manipulative Therapy.* NINDS Monograph 11. Washington, DC: US Department of Health, Education, and Welfare.

Mennell JM. Medical terminology. In *The Research Status of Spinal Manipulative Therapy.* NINDS Monograph 11. Washington, DC: US Department of Health, Education, and Welfare.

Mennell JM. The intervertebral disc & low backache. *N Z Med J.* 1947;46:40–44.

Mennell JM. *Joint Pain—Diagnosis and Treatment Using Manipulative Techniques.* Boston, Mass: Little, Brown and Company; 1964.

Mennell JM. Manipulation of the joints of the wrist. *The Journal of the Chartered Society of Physiotherapy.* 1971.

Mennell JM. Manipulation therapy for low back pain. In Bonica JJ et al, eds. *Advances in Pain Research and Therapy.* New York, NY: Raven Press; 1979.

Mennell JM. Manipulation and the treatment of low back pain. *Clin Orthop.* 1955;5.

Mennell JM. Manipulation and treatment of pain in the chest. *N Z Med J.* 1948; 48:586–598.

Mennell JM. Pain from mechanical dysfunction of synovial joints. Paper presented at the Proceedings of the 4th International Congress of Manual Medicine.

Mennell JM. The problem of the common case of low back pain. *Stamford Medical Bulletin.* 1951;9.

Mennell JM. Spray-stretch for the relief of pain from muscle spasm and myofascial trigger points. *J Am Podiat Med Assoc.* 1976;66:873–876.

Mennell JM. Survey of the anatomy of the spine. Prepared for the American Academy of Physical Medicine and Rehabilitation for review recertification syllabus.

Mennell JM. Therapeutic use of cold. *J Am Osteopath Assoc.* 1975;74:1146–1158.

Mennell JM. Understanding manipulative medicine in general practice. *J Manipulative Physiol Ther.* 1989;12:231–235.

Mennell JM, Smith D. The work values of veterans and some implications for educational therapy. *VA Newsletter for Research in Mental Health and Behavioral Sciences.* 1976;18.

Mennell JM, Zohn D. *Diagnosis and Physical Treatment of Musculoskeletal Pain.* Boston, Mass: Little, Brown and Company; 1976.

Still, AJ. Effects of lumbar lesions. AJ Still Research Institute. *Bulletin 5,* 1917.

Still, AJ. *Osteopathy.* 1897.

Still, AJ. The pathology of the vertebral lesion. AJ Still Research Institute. *Bulletin 4,* 1917.

Stoddard A. *Manual of Osteopathic Technique.* Hutchinson Medical Publications; 1959.

Travell J. *Office Hours: Day and Night.* New York, NY: The World Publishing Company; 1968.

Travell J, Simons D. *Myofascial Pain and Dysfunction: The Trigger Point Manual.* Baltimore, Md: Williams & Wilkins; 1983.

Wiles P. *Essentials of Orthopaedics.* London: J & A Churchill; 1959.

Wilkins R, ed. *Neurosurgery.* New York, NY: McGraw-Hill; 1987.

Index

Swallowing problems, forward head
    syndrome, 131–132
Sweat level, 71
Swollen joints, shoulder pain, 142
Symptoms, onset of, 39
Synovial capsule
    anatomical aspects, 10
    congenital abnormalities, 11
    inflammation of, 11
    metabolic disease, 11
    neoplasms, 11
    sensitivity of, 6
    trauma to, 10–11
Synovial fluid, 10, 24–25
    excess of, 42, 43
Synovial joint manipulation, 158–159
Syphilis, 142
System of body, approach to study of, 2
Systemic disease
    and joints, 11
    shoulder pain and, 147–148
    and trigger points, 112

T

Temperature, 44
Temperature of skin, 71
Temporomandibular joint pain, 137–136
    treatment approach, 138
Tendinitis, shoulder pain, 143
Tendons
    inflammation, 15
    musculotendinous junction, 15
    pathologic changes, 15
    tendinitis, 15
    trauma, 15
Tendon sheaths, pathologic changes, 16
Tennis elbow, 10
Tenosynovitis, of long head of biceps,
    143
Therapeutic manipulative techniques
    assisstive devices, 165–168
    See also Physical therapy
Thoracic kyphosis, increases, and chest
    wall pain, 136–137
Tietze's syndrome, 135
Traction, 161

Transcutaneous nerve stimulation, pain
    management, 153
Trauma
    avulsion fractures, 7
    bone, 8–9
    bursae, 17
    extrinsic trauma, 6
    hyaline cartilage, 9–10
    intrinsic trauma, 6
    ligaments, 11–12
    muscle, 13
    synovial capsule, 10–11
    tendons, 15
Travell's trigger points, 7, 13, 18, 125
Trigger points, 13, 14, 28, 111–118
    anterior scalene muscle, 118
    chest wall pain, 136
    deltoid muscle, 113
    diagnosis of, 112
    etiology of, 38–39, 112
    forward head syndrome, 130–131
    gluteus minimus muscle, 113
    jump sign, 112
    predictability of pain patterns, 112–113,
        114–118
    shoulder pain, 143–144
    spray and stretch, 159
    sternocleidomastoid muscle, 113
Tubercular joint, 25
Tuberculosis, 16, 43, 137, 142

U

Ultrasound, 157–158
Ultraviolet light, 142, 163–164

V

Vertebral percussion, importance of, 28
Visceral pain, 27, 35
Volkman's ischemic contracture, 13
Voluntary movements, examination of, 45

W

Walkers, 166
Wheelchairs, 166

About the Author

John McMillan Mennell, MD, is the foremost expert in the field of Manipulative Medicine. He has published numerous articles, books, and papers on all aspects of the field, and has done pioneering work on techniques of diagnosis. Dr. Mennell received a Master of Arts, Honoris Casua, in 1971 from the University of Pennsylvania. In 1976 he was awarded the Director's Commendation for Achievement in Equal Employment Opportunity from the Veterans Administration Hospital of Martinez, California. His work was honored in 1982 when the Mennell-Travell Lecture was inaugurated by the North American Academy of Manipulative Medicine. He was granted an honorary membership to the British Institute of Orthopaedic Medicine in 1983. In 1984 he won the ABC Knudson Award from the American Association of Rehabilitation Therapy, and in the same year delivered the Third Pierce Nelson Lecture for the California College of Podiatric Medicine. In 1986 he was awarded the Presidential Medal of Merit at the Eighth Congress of the International Federation of Manual Medicine in Madrid. And in 1989 he was awarded the P.T. Associates of Wharton, Texas Award of Merit. The Walter F. Patenge Medal of Public Service was awarded in 1989 to Dr. Mennell by Michigan State University, College of Osteopathic Medicine.